The Speech-Language Pathologist in Home Health Care

Cecil G. Betros, Jr., DSc, CCC-SLP
President and Chief Executive Officer
Communication Concepts and Consulting, Inc.
Birmingham, Alabama

AN ASPEN PUBLICATION®
Aspen Publishers, Inc.
Gaithersburg, Maryland
1999

The author has made every effort to ensure the accuracy of the information herein. However, appropriate information sources should be consulted, especially for new or unfamiliar procedures. It is the responsibility of every practitioner to evaluate the appropriateness of a particular opinion in the context of actual clinical situations and with due considerations to new developments. The author, editors, and the publisher cannot be held responsible for any typographical or other errors found in this book.

Library of Congress Cataloging-in-Publication Data

Betros, Cecil.
The speech-language pathologist in home health care / Cecil Betros, Jr.
p.   cm.
Includes bibliographical references and index.
ISBN 0-8342-0919-5
1. Speech disorders—Patients—Home care.   2. Speech therapy.   I. Title
RC428.5.B47   1999
616.85'506—dc21
98-48636
CIP

Orders: (800) 638-8437
Customer Service: (800) 234-1660

About Aspen Publishers • For more than 35 years, Aspen has been a leading professional publisher in a variety of disciplines. Aspen's vast information resources are available in both print and electronic formats. We are committed to providing the highest quality information available in the most appropriate format for our customers. Visit Aspen's Internet site for more information resources, directories, articles, and a searchable version of Aspen's full catalog, including the most recent publications: **http://www.aspenpublishers.com**
Aspen Publishers, Inc. • The hallmark of quality in publishing
Member of the worldwide Wolters Kluwer group.

Editorial Services: Kathy Litzenberg
Library of Congress Catalog Card Number: 98-48636
ISBN: 0-8342-0919-5

Printed in the United States of America

1 2 3 4 5

This book is dedicated to
Anne Kakoliris Betros, a wonderful
and supportive mother,
and
Sue Betros Graphos, Sam Graphos,
Ted Graphos, and Suzanne Graphos,
a loving family.

IN MEMORY OF
Cecil G. Betros, Sr.
James Michael Reese

Table of Contents

Preface

Communication disorders management in the home care setting involves the coordinated efforts of a number of specialists, primarily the speech-language pathologist, the physician, and a nurse. Speech, language, and swallowing rehabilitation in the home is directed at all medical, functional, organic, and psychological factors that combine to produce a communication deficit. Primary consideration is given to the devastating effects of the communication disorder for homebound patients. Listening and talking are the primary method of contact with the environment. When this vital link is impaired, the impact on the patient's emotional, social, and intellectual well-being can be overwhelming. Thus, the speech-language pathologist working in home health care must employ a dynamic process that transcends the traditional role of the typical speech-language pathologist's function in overall patient care.

The purpose of this book is not only to provide the clinician with a basic orientation to the practice of speech-language pathology in home health care but to provide by detailed example some new perspectives in meeting the diagnostic and treatment challenges that are particular to the home care environment. The philosophy of clinical practice in this book evolved from the author's 20 years' experience working in home health care. The book presents a comprehensive description of the distinctive nature of providing clinical speech, language, cognitive, and swallowing services to homebound individuals. The traditional role of the speech-language pathologist is discussed in terms of typically occurring practice methodologies and work settings. In addition, the role of the speech-language pathologist working in home care is discussed, and specific procedures are outlined. There is little documentation in the literature to substantiate the procedures outlined in this book, which derive strictly from the author's clinical experience. On the other hand, there is also no documentation to refute these suggested procedures. Specific case studies are also presented to illustrate the speech-language pathologist's role in relation to the homebound patient, showing its distinctive nature and its effectiveness in maximizing patient care. The appendixes at the end of the book contain specific forms and additional information. Appendix A contains the "Physician Certification and Plan of Treatment Requirements" as taken from the *Code of Federal Regulations,* Title 42. Appendix B is a sample referral form; Appendix C contains service codes for specific forms produced by the Health Care Financing Administration; Appendix D is a glossary of medical terms; and Appendix E is a list of general abbreviations.

In home care, traditional speech-language pathology methodologies and practices must be modified and/or expanded to include (1) acquiring the appropriate home care assessment tools to evaluate not only the patient but also the family dynamics; (2) assessing the adequacy of family/caregiver and informal care resources; (3) evaluating the efficacy of home care effort; (4) applying home care principles and guidelines appropriately; (5) knowing community resources and when to refer patients for such services; (6) being knowledgeable about home care technology, such as infection control procedures; (7) understanding about cost reimbursement policies in home health care; and (8) being a leader on the home care team.

Patient medical problems are a primary cause of communication deficits in the home health setting. The medical problem usually receives most of the attention and is the gateway or entry to the medical system. The physician, then, is the gatekeeper in controlling the services any given patient receives for any given condition. Speech-language pathologists must be skillful in educating physicians about the benefits of speech-language pathology. The speech-language pathologist must understand the world of medicine and consider how it operates. Speech-language pathologists should be familiar with not only medical terminology but also the function of each medical discipline. They must gain an understanding and a vision of their clinical practice, its relationship to medical care, and the expectations of the speech-language pathologist's role in home care.

Communication disorders management in the home is an arduous task but an exciting responsibility. The skills of the speech-language pathologist working in the home, combined with proper planning and patient care, can enable home care patients with communication disorders to make great strides toward increasing their ability to interact with others and to bridge the communication gap.

Acknowledgments

Many individuals have supported and assisted me throughout the years. First, I thank Dr. Loretta G. Brown, my friend and mentor not only through graduate school but also during my career, for believing in me for all these years.

I thank Myra J. Downs, RN, MSN, for showing me the way in home health care for the past 22 years. Thanks to you, Myra, this book was developed and written.

I greatly appreciate the support and encouragement of my staff and colleagues during the writing of this book. I especially thank Laura Waldrip, RN, MSN.

Finally, I thank Michael Lee, who inspired the design on the cover of this book, and Dwayne Johnson and Vicki Ray, who typed the manuscript.

PART I

The Home Health Model

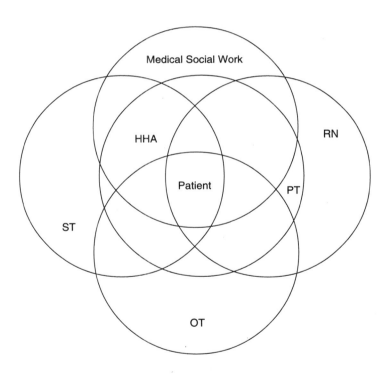

CHAPTER 1

Introduction and an Overview of Home Health Care

HOME CARE DEVELOPMENT

The informal, sympathetic care of the sick in their homes by relatives and friends has a long history. The delivery of systematic nursing care in the home, that is, care based on the best available knowledge of the natural history of disease, is a much more recent undertaking and is a result of Florence Nightingale's program of secular scientific education for nurses (Smith, 1983). William Rathbone supported philanthropic projects aimed at the sick poor in Liverpool, and Nightingale nurses ran and staffed some of the projects (Woodham-Smith, 1970).

The notion of delivering skilled nursing services to the sick and poor was also developing in the United States. Philanthropists in this country provided funds for the start-up of voluntary organizations, forerunners of the visiting nurse associations (VNAs), and trained nurses were hired to deliver home nursing services similar to services in England. As local health departments developed and expanded in the early years of the twentieth century, health officers in charge of these "official" agencies added nurses to their staffs. One of the nursing responsibilities was the delivery of services in the home. By the middle part of this century, a number of these voluntary and official agencies had combined their resources to varying degrees, streamlined their operations, and thus decreased overhead, costs, and service duplication. Such organizations became known as *combination agencies.*

In 1947, another innovative service mode was instituted. E.M. Bluestone, a physician at Montefiore Hospital in The Bronx, New York, introduced the notion of hospital-based home care. Patients discharged from the hospital were entitled to a wide range of nursing, social, and other related services, all delivered in their own homes (Cherkasky, 1949). Such an arrangement, a health care institution operating a department of home care, is no longer limited to hospitals. Rehabilitation centers and skilled nursing facilities also offer home health service departments.

These departments of home care are referred to as *institution-based agencies*. In contrast, agencies that are not part of an institution are referred to as *free-standing agencies*.

RECENT HISTORY

By the mid-1960s, there were approximately 1,200 free-standing agencies delivering home health services (Mundinger, 1983), and most of the services were paid for by donations through organizations such as local community chests or by the recipients of the care. The passage of Medicare and, to a lesser extent, Medicaid in the mid-1960s spurred the growth of the home health industry, because these federal insurance programs ensure a stable source of income for the agencies eligible to participate in them. The growth of the private agency, another type of agency for the delivery of home health services, was further stimulated in 1982 when Congress and the Health Care Financing Administration opened up home health care to the for-profit sector for Medicare reimbursement.

Although the increase in the number of hospital-based home care agencies has been steady, the growth spurt between 1984 and 1993 was due to the implementation of the prospective payment system for hospitals by Congress. Increasing numbers of acute care hospitals have been diversifying to broaden their revenue base, and home health care has been one of the areas targeted for this diversification (Ginzbert, Balinsky, & Ostow, 1984). Noncertified agencies, such as homemaker/home health aide agencies, provide a variety of services under contract with certified agencies. The number of noncertified agencies is unknown, but the assumption is that there are at least as many noncertified as certified agencies (Moyer, 1986).

This chapter describes the similarities and differences among voluntary, official, and private home health agencies. They are similar in administrative structure and sources of funding. The major differences are the agencies' positioning for tax purposes and financial control or ownership.

FINANCIAL CONCERNS

The term *not for profit* is a designation that exempts organizations from taxation on profits or excess income under Section 501 of the Internal Revenue Code of 1954. This excess is put back into the organization, and no part of the net earnings can be used for the private benefit of owners, partners, or shareholders. Thus, a voluntary organization, such as a VNA or a community-owned hospital, is usually not for profit. If a not-for-profit organization wants to engage in activities intended to make a profit or surplus that is shared or distributed, it would have to form holding companies or separate corporate entities to deal with those profit-making actions. Many VNAs and hospitals are doing this in today's competitive market.

The terms *for profit* and *profit making* are also designations for tax purposes. Agencies with these designations are called *proprietary agencies,* and they are not eligible for tax exemption under Section 501 of the Internal Revenue Code. It must be remembered that such designations for tax purposes are not true differentiations of financial status. For example, all business organizations (voluntary and private) must make profits or at least have income equal to expenses to continue to exist.

Terms such as *government agency, nongovernmental, private, church affiliated*, and the like all refer to control of ownership, not to positioning for tax purposes. The health department is an example of an official government agency created to perform specified public functions, such as drinking water purification, and services, such as public health nursing. It is maintained from revenues such as taxes and fees collected from the people who benefit from its services or functions. Within this context, therefore, a community-owned agency is usually not for profit, but a privately owned organization such as a home health agency could be either for profit or not for profit.

SCOPE OF HOME CARE

Home care is one of many service components in the arena of long-term care, although it is not limited to long-term care. Other service components of long-term care include skilled nursing facilities and programs for substance abusers and for persons who are developmentally, occupationally, and physically disabled. In other words, many different age and population groups require continuing care.

Within this long-term care context, however, the phrase *home health care* refers both to the range of in-home services provided to chronically ill people over a long period of time and to the Medicare-reimbursed home-based services that are primarily for acutely ill older persons and are skilled, short term, and intermittent (Moyer, 1986). Regardless of how home health is defined, however, nursing care is the foundation of the entire system.

RANGE OF HOME HEALTH AGENCIES

The Medicare Conditions of Participation for home health agencies define a home health agency as "a public agency or private organization, primarily engaged in providing skilled nursing services and other therapeutic services" (Health Care Financing Administration, 1996). Certified home health agencies must have a professional advisory committee, a requirement for participation in the Medicare program. This group of professional persons establishes policies and governs the services provided by the home health agency. Appropriate professional discipline representation is required, with a minimum of one physician and one registered nurse. In recent years, consumer representation has been strongly encouraged by the Medicare auditing agencies. This committee must review the agency's policies on an annual basis and provide an advisory function on a timely, regular, and planned basis.

Government Agencies

Government (official) home health agencies are "created and given their power through statutes enacted by legislators" (Stewart, 1979, p. 25). Home health services are frequently provided by the nursing division of state or local health departments. The organizational structure within the nursing divisions varies. Some agencies opt to have public health nurses include their home health clients in their overall public health caseload. Other government agencies choose to form home health teams within their nursing departments whose primary function is to provide home health services. Local health departments may have a combination of both public health nurses and home health team nurses providing home health services.

In addition to home health services, government agencies usually provide services such as disease prevention, home health promotion, communicable disease investigation, environmental health, maternal-child health, and family planning.

Fiscal responsibility for the government home health agency rests with the city, county, or state government units or a combination of such organizations. The overall city, county, or state budget restrictions can directly influence the provision of health services in a particular area. Home health caseloads of government agencies frequently include a disproportionate number of indigent patients, since the agency cannot refuse services on the basis of ability to pay. There is a growing trend throughout the United States for government agencies to decrease or eliminate the provision of home health services. This trend may be due to the indigent client issue as well as other politically motivated issues that influence the types of health services provided by a government agency. Increasingly, government agencies are focusing on the more traditional public health services, so in the future there may be a decline of government-sponsored Medicare-certified home health agencies.

Voluntary Agencies

Home health agencies that do not depend on state and local tax revenues but are financed primarily with nontax funds—such as donations, endowments, United Way contributions, and third-party insurance payouts (Medicare, Medicaid, and Blue Cross)—are referred to as *voluntary agencies*. An example is the VNA. Voluntary agencies are governed by a board of directors of interested individuals, who are frequently respected members of the surrounding community or service area. These agencies are considered community-based agencies because they provide services within a fairly well-defined geographic location or community. In recent years, however, traditional VNA boundaries have become less distinct as a result of increased competition for clients. In the past, voluntary agencies' client base included virtually all the home health patients within their own catchment area, but the growth of proprietary and institution-based home health agencies has now eroded their traditional referral base. The relationship between neighboring VNAs has turned from cooperation to competition in many instances.

Private Agencies

Private home health agencies can be for-profit or not-for-profit organizations. Some proprietary (for-profit) agencies participate in the Medicare home health program as part of national chains and are administered through corporate head-quarters.

Although revenues are generated by some proprietary agencies through third-party payers such as Medicare and Blue Cross, other proprietaries rely on private pay clients. These private pay agencies offer services such as private duty nursing to both acutely and chronically ill patients, whereas most Medicare-certified pro-viders primarily provide services to patients who have had a recent acute change in their medical condition. Private pay agency services are often on an extended-hours basis (2 to 24 hours) rather than on a per-visit basis (O'Malley, 1986). Many such agencies also provide hospital staffing services.

Institution-Based Agencies

Home health agencies operating as departments in sponsoring health care orga-nizations are certified under Medicare and hold a separate provider number, but they are governed by the sponsoring organization's board of trustees or directors.

In the past, home health services provided by institution-based providers con-sisted of intensive-level services intended for those clients requiring multi-discipline services and supplies. The case mix of today's institution-based agen-cies reflects the change to a more balanced caseload in which patients require differing degrees of services. The principal source of referrals for these agencies is the inpatient population of the facility, with discharge planning/social services being the case finder of potential home health clients.

The philosophy of the institution-based agency usually coincides with that of the sponsoring organization. Good continuity of care is frequently cited by these agencies as their primary advantage over other types of home health agencies (Stewart, 1979). This continuity can be sold to the medical staff of the institution by promoting the fact that the home care is coordinated by persons familiar with the physicians and the institution.

A fiscal advantage of institution-based home health providers is that Medicare allows the inclusion of a percentage of administrative and general overhead in the calculation of the visit costs. The Medicare home health reimbursement system once also recognized the higher costs of office space in hospitals and permitted an add-on amount in the calculation of the visit costs, but this add-on was eliminated as a result of tax reform legislation of 1993 (National Association for Home Care, 1993). Another advantage enjoyed by the institution-based home health agency is the ability to draw from the resources of the other departments of the facility for service provision as well as for formal and informal consultation services.

Hospice

The National Hospice Organization (1984) defines hospice as an agency in which "services are provided by a medically supervised interdisciplinary team of professionals and volunteers" for terminally ill patients. Hospices can be institution based, owned by or affiliated with a certified home health agency, or independently owned. There are variations among home care hospice programs in their structure and staffing, but all profess to foster the provision of palliative and supportive services to the patient as well as to the family after the patient's demise. This service is unique to hospice agencies because other home health agencies' services end upon the death of the patient.

The hospice concept was imported from Britain to the United States at New Haven in the mid-1970s, and there are now more than 1,400 programs. Hospice services are reimbursed by many health insurance plans, such as Blue Cross/ Blue Shield, as well as by the home hospice service Medicare benefit provided in the Tax Equity and Fiscal Responsibility Act of 1982 (National Hospice Organization, 1984). Many hospice agencies have chosen to obtain Medicare certification because of the improved reimbursement schedule outlined by recent regulations.

Homemaker/Home Health Aide Agencies

Agencies providing homemaker and home health aide services are frequently private agencies in which patients or private insurance policies pay for the home care services (Stewart, 1979). These agencies can provide home health aides who are Medicare certified; that is, they have completed a Medicare-approved home health aide course of study (75 hours in length) and/or passed competency evaluation procedures. With these certified aides, homemaker/health aide agencies are able to contract with Medicare-certified home health agencies, which, in turn, are reimbursed by Medicare for the home health aide services. The Medicare-certified agency pays the homemaker/home health aide agency directly on an hourly basis.

Such contracts are lucrative because they are guaranteed income for the home-maker/home health agency.

The distinction between homemakers and home health aides can at times be difficult to ascertain because both functions are often provided by a single employee. Homemakers function primarily as housecleaners, whereas the principal duties of home health aides are in the area of personal care, such as bathing. More complex services, such as range of motion exercises, can be performed by the home health aide after proper instruction by a registered nurse.

Homemaker/home health aide agencies are required to ensure that their staff complete 12 hours of inservice programs per year to meet Medicare standards. In addition, on-site performance evaluations are conducted by professionals, such as registered nurses.

OTHER HOME HEALTH CARE PROVIDERS

In addition to home health agencies, home care is provided by home health services such as durable medical equipment companies, high-technology services companies (which provide ventilators, total parenteral nutrition, etc.), and home telephone reassurance programs. Home health care reflects most strongly the impact of Medicare and Medicaid, the government-funded medical programs that began in the 1960s. Nevertheless, public health initiatives, private insurance benefit regulation, and newly emerging health problems contribute to a constantly changing picture. The home health care services secured in a particular case ultimately depend on the complex interactions among patient, family, and community needs; patient and professionals' goals; and the payment sources available to fund service organizations such as home health care agencies.

Four prominent national organizations involved in home health care provision—the Council of Home Health Agencies and Community Health Services of the National League for Nursing, the National Homecaring Council (formerly known as the National Home Care Council), the National Association of Home Health Agencies, and the Assembly of Outpatient and Home Care Institutions of the American Hospital Association—provide a formal definition of home health care:

> Home health services is that component of comprehensive health care whereby services are provided to individuals and families in their places of residence for the purpose of promoting, maintaining, or restoring health or minimizing the effects of illness and disability. Service appropriate to the needs of the individual patient and family is planned, coordinated, and made available by an agency or institution, organized for the delivery of health care through the use of employed staff, contrac-

tual arrangements, or a combination of administrative patterns. (McNamara, 1982, p. 61)

DESCRIPTION OF HOME HEALTH CARE

Home health care begins with the patient, the individual identified as requiring home nursing or therapy services. Although this identified individual is the focus of the home health care services, professional goals for patient development are implemented in the context of family and community. The family, neighbors, and other members of the patient's informal support system generally provide the 24-hour care and support during the patient's period of illness or dependence. Formal services from home health agencies or the community's social service network can only supplement what family and friends provide. The more dependent the patient, the greater the skill and commitment demanded from the informal caregiving system. If family and friends are unable to provide adequate care, and if the patient requires more intensive services than those available from the home health agency, consideration of skilled nursing facilities or sheltered care placement becomes critical.

Because of the interactive reliance on informal supports in home health care, it is most practical to define the family in a flexible manner. Traditional definitions of family that include only close biological relatives are inadequate and can limit caregiving resources. In practice, family must include anyone whom the patient so identifies. In addition to the nuclear family, persons included may be distant relatives, a boarder who has lived in the home for years, close friends, or neighbors who perceive a mutual obligation with the patient. This flexible definition of family increases the pool of available helpers for the dependent client but also requires that nursing and other home health care workers incorporate the needs of this extended family system into plans of care. In providing care, nurses must consider both the learning needs of support system members and the psychosocial supports required to maintain their caregiving roles. It is not enough simply to instruct. Meeting the needs of the support system requires complex coordination and problem solving as well.

The patient's community may facilitate or detract from the provision of professional care and the fulfillment of home health care service objectives. Communities vary from densely concentrated urban neighborhoods to sprawling suburban towns to lonesome rural back roads. Although a client may be isolated from supports in any environment, the concentration of people and services, the availability of transportation, and the proximity and diversity of pharmacy and grocery services make a quantitative difference in the challenges faced by home health care patients and families.

The community, and the membership of the patient and the family within it, has further effects on the patient and family system and their presenting needs for home health care. Patients' and families' socioeconomic background and class status frequently influence their access to care. The family's cultural and ethnic background influences its expectations for health and health care services and its ability to meet those needs within the U.S. health care system. Individuals, families, and communities have particular ways of defining health, illness, and dying that home health care professionals must recognize and address. For example, many religious groups have prohibitions of which formal caregivers should be aware. Home care professionals must acquire the ability to practice within cultural parameters.

Health professionals are usually trained to hospital goals and values, and they find differences at every step in home care. The most obvious difference cannot be minimized: The home in all its many variations has replaced the hospital. Rather than patients adapting to the foreign environment of the hospital, it is home health care providers themselves who must adapt to the family, community, and home environment. Home care skilled providers are liaisons, expert consultants who adapt complex treatment plans to homes. This may involve, for example, obtaining equipment, making referrals to other services, or negotiating with physicians to alter medication or nutritional intake programs.

INITIATION OF HOME HEALTH CARE SERVICES

Home health patients are visited by home care agency personnel after referrals are made for the patient's care. Referrals may originate from the patient, the family, a community social service agency, a local physician, or almost anyone else. Many home care referrals are initiated by hospital staff, such as nurses, social workers, or discharge planners. These referrals are made to home health agencies from hospitals when patient needs for continuing care are identified during the hospitalization or while the patient is under care at an ambulatory clinic or emergency department. Additional referrals are received from nursing homes, community clinics, physicians' offices, area agencies on aging, and social work agencies.

The referral to home health care services includes the patient's demographic information, family contacts, diagnoses, medications, and proposed treatment measures ordered by the physician. Professional disciplines to be provided to the patient are specified. This referral is often not overly complex and generally focuses on the basic, immediate needs of the patient. Even so, it is most helpful for the referral to include patient data such as a brief medical and surgical history, recent laboratory findings, baseline vital sign readings, and history and course of the present illness. Because the patient's social context suggests both needs and limitations of care, knowledge of patient and family strengths and weaknesses pertaining to the illness and home management will provide a head start for home health agency professionals.

For Medicare home care referrals, it is important to consider patients' functional abilities. Are the patients substantially confined to the home? Several contemporary payment sources for home care require that patients receiving services be homebound. Although the definition of homebound status has varied, it has generally been interpreted to mean that the patient's health and functional impairment is so great that he or she is unable to leave the home to seek health services. Additional variables, such as the presence or absence of a safe patient environment and a reliable caregiver, may also influence whether services can be provided in the home.

The organizations that provide home health care may be voluntary agencies, such as VNAs; proprietary agencies; official health departments; social service agencies; or hospital-based home care departments. Whatever the organizational structure, most agencies visit postacute home health care patients within 24 hours of the initial referral. The first visit will probably be the most complex of the entire service period. During this admission visit, the nurse conducts an assessment and evaluation of the patient and family, assesses the environmental milieu, analyzes the impact of the disease(s) on the patient, identifies functional impairments of the patient, determines the patient's knowledge of and adherence to the prescribed treatment for the disease, and identifies patient/family desires for care and eventual goals. Nurses establish the groundwork for needed services and ensure the safety of the patient until the next home care visit. Physical therapists or speech therapists may also take primary responsibility for a home health care case. Active participation of patients and families in the goals of treatment and plans of care is sought and utilized to the fullest extent.

Patients receive services for varying periods of time, from a single visit to multiple visits over several weeks, months, or even years. Visit patterns are usually controlled by reimbursement regulations, resulting in varying patterns of care controlled from outside the patient-provider nexus. Under Medicare, visits continue until the patient's skilled care needs are met. This period is usually short, most often less than two months. Under Medicare, patients requiring technical interventions such as dressing changes or indwelling urinary catheter management may have intermittent services over several years. Case management systems, such as those used in health maintenance organizations, are often the most restrictive. For example, sometimes they allow only two or three visits to complete all instruction to a new insulin-dependent diabetic patient. Other reimbursement sources address distinct requirements, resulting in different patterns of care. For example, in maternal-child programs, nursing visits may be spaced at long intervals as long as chronic conditions are controlled, but hospice program visits may be frequent (sometimes daily), particularly for patients in late, terminal stages of disease.

Home care professionals work with patients and families to establish plans of care that address the long-term goals of the case, working toward incremental change during each visit. The home health care nurse uses many resources to facilitate patient and family progress. Services of additional multidisciplinary team members, such as the physical therapist, occupational therapist, social worker, speech therapist, and home health aide, may be used for the patient's benefit. If rehabilitation goals predominate, physical therapy or speech therapy may be the only discipline providing service. Home health care professionals communicate with the patient's physician to coordinate the treatment plan with changes in the patient's status, for example, progress in rehabilitation, difficulty in wound healing, or persistent challenges of the terminal phase of illness.

The home health care team relies heavily on ongoing services provided by the community's formal support network as well as on the family's own informal support system. Ongoing support systems are essential to prepare the patient for discharge from home health care and to provide needed services when skilled care through the home health agency is terminated. The nurse or other professional will make, or suggest that the patient or family make, appropriate referrals to formal care networks. The nurse will also seek to develop and support informal systems based in the family, neighborhood, or social groups.

Although actual outcomes vary significantly among patients and families, case discharge usually occurs when the patient has met the goals of care. Some patients progress easily and completely to meet mutually set goals for care; others may achieve only partial outcomes. The patient is prepared for discharge throughout the whole period of home health care provision by being taught the skills required to resume independent management of health care needs. At discharge, the nurse or other home health care provider notifies the physician and other involved services that the case is closed. Discharged cases are reopened when patients are referred for new problems or exacerbation of health problems addressed previously.

REASONS FOR THE GROWTH IN HOME HEALTH CARE

Not only has home health care expanded, but it also holds potential for future expansion as a result of expected changes in the contemporary sociopolitical situation and in economic forces, which together provide the environment for home health care. Changing patterns of disease and population, emerging economic reimbursement mechanisms, and changing social values draw together to construct the contemporary home health care delivery system.

The change in the distribution of disease since the turn of the twentieth century provides the first factor in the growth of home health care. Improved scientific knowledge of disease agents, regular immunizations, the availability of antibiotics, provision of basic nutrition to most people, pasteurization of milk, and other factors have decreased the risk of developing and dying from disease threats such as tuberculosis, severe diarrhea illnesses, cholera, and many others. In place of acute illnesses, chronic illnesses are now the primary causes of death in the United States. These illnesses, such as hypertension, cardiac disease, pulmonary disease, and diabetes, have a long period of development leading to irreversible changes in the body and frequently permanent impairment of the individual's functional abilities. Although early intervention may limit the exacerbation of chronic disease, affected individuals generally experience long periods of debilitation necessitating rehabilitation, during which they may fail to regain their previous abilities. The health care delivery system is faced with making policy decisions about people for whom illness and disease are irreversible, degenerative, and function impairing. Long-term chronic illness reduces individual and family resources and decreases financial ability to pay privately for needed services. It will be a challenge to society to develop systems that are efficient in meeting patient needs and effective in controlling overall costs. Home care has shown promise in being the alternative of choice to meet this large and growing need.

A second and related impact on the growth of home health care is the change in the U.S. population distribution. The nation is growing older as a whole. Although in 1900 only 4.1 percent of Americans were older than 65 years, by 1984 this had tripled to 11.9 percent, a change in real numbers from 3.1 million to 28.0 million (American Association of Retired Persons, 1985). This increase in the population over age 65 is interrelated with the increased prevalence of chronic illnesses in the distribution of disease. With decreased mortality due to acute illnesses in the younger population, more individuals are living into their later years, the time at which chronic illness is more likely to appear. In addition, better treatment of complications of old age and chronic illness means that even with serious disease people tend to live longer than before.

Complicating the population trend toward longer life have been changes in the social behavior of families. Changing distribution of employment, economic recession, and improved transportation have dispersed families across the country more than ever before. When older persons require assistance, they may have few relatives living close by who can help them. Changing patterns of female employment, which have increased the percentage of women in the work force, have simultaneously reduced the number of female family members available for full-time care of the chronically ill. As a result of all these structural changes in the family, care of impaired older persons may need to be increasingly a social and government responsibility.

A third factor in the growth of home health care, and also an effect of the increase in chronic illness prevalence, has been the expansion of rehabilitative services for those at home with chronic illness. Rehabilitation is a long-term process requiring adaptation of the impaired individual back into the home environment.

This adaptation may require diverse professional services. Home health care has expanded its use of physical therapy, occupational therapy, and speech therapy in home rehabilitation efforts. Social work also has a place in the care of the homebound individual. When individuals require a diversity of services, overall use of home health care increases.

Changing reimbursement patterns have had such a profound effect on the outline of services provided under home health care that reimbursement is said to set the direction for home health care. A look at the history of the practice field substantiates this position, but changing reimbursement has had an especially strong impact on the rise in home health care since the passage of Medicare and Medicaid home care coverage with the Social Security amendments of 1965 and the first services offered in 1966. The Medicare focus is on short-term home care management. Further, Medicare reimbursement has made home health care a profitable venture for proprietary agencies and hospitals, and thus the number of agencies, both with and without certificates of need, has multiplied. Competition has thus far led to growth, but it has also raised questions of quality assurance because of the lack of specific training in home health care skills in the new agencies.

The search for health care cost containment has also encouraged the growth of home health care. The changes in Medicare reimbursement for hospitalization toward a prospective payment system, popularly known as the *diagnosis-related group (DRG) system,* have given fiscal encouragement to limit the length of acute hospitalizations. A result has been the discharge home or to nursing homes of individuals who in other times may have remained in the acute care institution. The phrase "sicker and quicker" has been used to describe the situation of those released to home care under this program. Increased acuity of home care patients implies more frequent skilled visits, more time-consuming visits as a result of increased complexity, and more patients at greater risk for decompensation and rehospitalization. A shift of care from acute institutions to home care is the foundation for still further changes in home health care.

The optimistic belief that cost containment motives will increase home health care use is tempered by at least two different problems. First, the desire for overall cost containment in health services, instead of increasing reimbursement to encourage hospital discharge, is paradoxically curtailing home care services offered to the patient. Medicare intermediaries, in particular, have attempted to strictly limit the categories of clients reimbursed under Medicare regulations of skilled care, intermittent services, and homebound status. Second, some experts have questioned whether the real total cost of patient care has been identified for use in comparisons with costs of acute hospital care. Lost income to the family and caregiver, cost of physical maintenance of the home, and other informal costs have not usually been part of the comparison equation.

Earlier acute discharge combined with increased availability of sophisticated biomedical equipment to home care leads to another factor increasing home care. Complex services once rarely seen in the home, such as renal hemodialysis treatment, ventilator therapy, and infusion therapy of many types, are more frequently an option for patients who prefer to be at home rather than endure long-term hospital stays. Simplified technology, effective teaching of patients' caregivers, and efficient supplier networks providing diverse equipment have allowed complex care to be given in the home environment.

A final area affecting the growth in home health care is the question of quality of life. Older and chronically ill patients would prefer to remain in their independent living situations rather than be institutionalized, for instance, in a nursing home. Many families view institutionalization and separation of family members negatively. Some cultural and ethnic groups are especially reluctant to treat chronically ill and older individuals in this manner. A desire for self-care as part of significant long-term changes in popular philosophy has also supported increases in home health care. Despite these significant trends in societal values, the necessary social and economic supports for patients and family caregivers involved in long-term home care are rarely provided.

Home health care has become an essential aspect of health care. The challenge will be to draw from home health care's past, anticipate its future potential, and provide effective services to contemporary patients and families.

CURRENT TRENDS AND DEFINITIONS

"Home is where the heart is," whether home is a house, an apartment, a residents' club, a mansion, or a shanty. To most Americans, home is emphatically not a hospital, nursing home, rest home, or sanitarium. There is a widespread feeling that home is for healthy people, while institutions are places for sick people. Nevertheless, in recent times, people diagnosed as ill have been removed from their homes, where they felt most comfortable, and treated in unfamiliar and often frightening surroundings. Only recently has the trend begun to reverse, but the "homecoming" of health-related in-home services has been both praised and criticized.

More babies are being born at home, and more people are dying there. Acute care services, now available at home for persons discharged early from institutions, are equally effective when used to prolong the institutionalization. Chronically ill, aged, and disabled patients are being helped to regain and retain their independence with the assistance of home health providers. Meeting the different health needs of all home care clients—young and old patients, urban and rural dwellers, and those who live alone as well those who live with others—is the goal of home health care services.

Home health services are that part of comprehensive health care that is provided to individuals in their places of residence for the purpose of promoting, maintaining, or restoring health, or of minimizing the effects of illness and disability. Home health care is a unique modality within the continuum of the health care delivery system. Like institutional or ambulatory health care, home health care is one of several methods of delivering health care services. For certain persons, it is the best and most appropriate method of care—just as hospitalization, a visit to the physician's office, or a "rest cure" at a health spa is best for others. Unfortunately, home health is sometimes incorrectly discussed only as a less costly alternative to hospital care. Home health is not simply an alternative to institutionalization, and it is definitely not "cut rate" or "second best" health care.

In past years, institutionalized care has been an accepted standard for health care. Rapid technological advances in the medical field, particularly in the development of "miracle surgery," have fostered the belief that the best health care is provided in large medical facilities offering the latest in machines and technology. It has been presumed that a person receiving a multitude of services in an institutional setting was receiving good care. With the new emphasis on holistic, humanistic health care, consumers and providers are now questioning those assumptions and seeking additional methods for delivering health care. A major factor for this movement is dissatisfaction with the old, cold, technical, and impersonal disease approach to health care and a preference for the more personal holistic approach.

Home health services can be provided before or after institutionalization. Many community-based health care providers emphasize preinstitutional services in the belief that effective home care can prevent or substantially delay unwanted institutional care (Stewart, 1979). Home care can also be seen as a means of facilitating early patient discharge, an idea that is particularly attractive since the development of DRGs and cost-conscious prepay group health plans. Both preinstitutional and postinstitutional care are important needs that the home health industry can fill in the total schema of the health care system.

In fact, it is most logical to consider the home as the primary site of health care delivery, with the institution as the alternative setting. The unique place of home care within the health care system was a major theme expressed at nationwide hearings as early as 1976 (Department of Health, Education and Welfare, 1976). Area studies at that time showed that 25 percent to 40 percent of persons in institutions may have been improperly placed (Morris, 1974). These people could function equally well or better in the home environment if minimum supportive services were available to them.

Since 1980, home health care has been a rapidly growing field and is one of the most dynamic segments of today's health care industry. Factors contributing to the growth in home health care include the following: the aging population, the growing number of children identified as needing home care, the pressure on hospitals to decrease cost by reducing the length of stays and limiting the number of beds, government and private efforts to contain cost, technological advances, and consumer needs or preferences for receiving services within the home (American Speech-Language-Hearing Association [ASHA], 1988).

Halammandaris (1991) reported that in 1990 the health care field led all U.S. industries in job growth, with a 7.7 percent increase. Within the general health care category, however, home care registered a job growth of 19.2 percent in 1990. All indications are that the growth rate will continue for several years (Batey & Horton, 1992).

The early 1990s were home health's "glory days." In 1998, however, home care faced reduced reimbursement from Medicare and a prospective payment system due to begin in 1999. In addition, Outcome and Assessment Information Set (OASIS) standards developed by the Health Care Financing Administration are on the horizon. Home care has become a turbulent industry. The industry is under extreme pressure to reduce costs and improve outcomes. How these changes will affect the practice of speech-language pathology in the future remains a mystery. Speech-language pathologists working in home health care today must spend a large amount of time reviewing and examining upcoming changes in the home health care industry.

The increased use of home health care and the potential for further expansion of the field of speech-language pathology result from economic forces and the many changes in the contemporary sociopolitical situation, which together provide the environment for home health care. According to Harris (1997), changing patterns of disease and population, emerging economic reimbursement mechanisms, and changing social values draw together to construct the contemporary home health delivery system. For the most part, this statement is true, but for the speech-language pathologist working in home health in 1998, this may not be the entire picture.

So how does speech-language pathology fit into this ever-changing home health environment? Management of the patient with a communication disorder is determined by the functional and/or organic nature of the problem. Most authorities (Batey & Horton, 1992; ASHA, 1988; Swanson & Albrecht, 1993) agree that disorders of communication require a total approach to remediation using a number of specialists in addition to the speech-language pathologist. Speech, language, and swallowing rehabilitation is directed at all the medical, functional, and/or organic and psychological factors that combine to produce a communication deficit. Work, interaction with the family and friends, and participation in community activities and routine activities of daily living all require the ability to communicate. When communication is impaired, individuals' ability to understand and express their thoughts, needs, and feelings associated with each of these life experiences is also impaired.

CONCLUSION

The categories of home health agencies have changed in the past two decades, and the future may bring new organizational structures that are now beginning to evolve. The beginning of the prospective payment system requires improved patient outcomes that must be achieved with limited financial resources and limited visits, leading to a new era in the provision of home health care services for all disciplines concerned. New alliances, formed mostly out of economic necessity, may continue to blur the distinction among the types of home health agencies and their ability to provide care to patients, thus creating even more complexities with which the home care speech-language pathologist must cope.

Among all the change, the speech-language pathologist and other health care workers must keep in mind that for the homebound patient, a communication disability is a serious problem. For such an individual, listening and talking become the primary method of contact within the environment. When this vital link is impaired, the impact on the patient's emotional, social, and intellectual well-being can be overwhelming. Thus, the speech-language pathologist working in home health care must have experience in using a multidynamic process. Home health care also transcends traditional roles of the speech-language pathologist in overall patient care. In addition, traditional treatment programs and strategies must be modified to meet the multifaceted needs of the homebound patient.

REFERENCES

American Association of Retired Persons. (1985). *A profile of older Americans.* Washington, DC: Author.

American Speech-Language-Hearing Association. (1988). The guidelines for the delivery of speech-language pathology in home care. *ASHA, 30* (Suppl. 3), 77–79.

Batey, J.M., & Horton, A.M. (1992). Homecare: The future is now. *ASHA,* 45–47.

Cherkasky, M. (1949). The Montefiore Hospital home care program. *American Journal of Public Health, 39,* 163–166.

Department of Health, Education and Welfare. (1976). *Home health care report of the regional public hearings* (DHEW Publication No. 76-135). Washington, DC: U.S. Government Printing Office.

Ginzbert, E., Balinsky, W., & Ostow, M. (1984). *Home health care.* Totowa, NJ: Rowman & Allanheld.

Halammandaris, J. (1991). The power of caring. *Caring Magazine, X*(10), 4–10.

Harris, M.D. (1997). *Home health administration.* Gaithersburg, MD: Aspen Publishers.

Health Care Financing Administration. (1996). *Conditions of participation. Home health agencies.* (Transmittal 277, Publication 11). Washington, DC: U.S. Government Printing Office.

McNamara, E. (1982). Home care: Hospitals discover comprehensive home care. *Hospitals, 56,* 60–66.

Morris, R. (1974). The development of parallel services for the elderly and disabled: Financial dimensions. *Gerontologist, 14,* 14–19.

Moyer, N. (1986). Public policy, politics, and home health care. *Home Health Care Nurse, 4,* 1–12.

Mundinger, M.O. (1983). *Home care controversy.* Gaithersburg, MD: Aspen Publishers.

National Association for Home Care (NAHC). (1993). NAHC Report No. 528. Washington, DC: Author.

National Hospice Organization. (1984). *The basics of hospice.* Arlington, VA: Author.

O'Malley, S.T. (1986). Reimbursement issues. In S. Stuart-Siddal (Ed.), *Home health care nursing. Administrative and clinical perspectives* (pp. 23–82). Gaithersburg, MD: Aspen Publishers.

Smith, J.A. (1983). *The idea of health.* New York: Teachers College Press.

Stewart, J.E. (1979). *Home health care.* St. Louis, MO: Mosby.

Swanson, J.M., & Albrecht, M. (1993). *Community health nursing.* Philadelphia: W.B. Saunders Company.

Woodham-Smith, C. (1970). *Florence Nightingale: 1820–1910.* London: Fontana.

SUGGESTED READING

Berg, B., et al. (1970). Assessing the health care needs of the aged. *Health Services Response, 5,* 36–59.

Cunningham, R.M., Jr. (1985). The evolution of hospice. Part 1. *Hospitals, 59,* 124–126.

In-home speech-language pathology services. (1988). *Caring Magazine, 19,* 16–17.

Miller, R.M., & Groher, M.E. (1990). *Medical speech pathology.* Rockville, MD: Aspen Publishers.

Paden, E.P. (1970). *A history of the American Speech and Hearing Association, 1925–1958.* Washington, DC: American Speech and Hearing Association.

Perkins, W.H. (1977). *Speech pathology: An applied behavioral science.* St. Louis, MO: CV Mosby.

Schruthfield, F.D., & Freeborn, D.K. (1971). Estimation of need, utilization, and costs of personal care homes and health services. *HSMA Health Report, 86,* 372–376.

Stanbert, T.E. (1977). A national study of United States hospital speech pathology services (Report No. 1). *ASHA, 19,* 160–163.

U.S. Bureau of the Census. (1980). *Characteristics of rural and farm-related population* (Publication No. PC 80-2.9). Washington, DC: Author.

Van Riper, C. (1971). *Speech correction: Principles and methods.* Englewood Cliffs, NJ: Prentice Hall.

CHAPTER 2

Scope of Home Health Speech-Language Pathology Practice

THE PRINCIPLES OF REHABILITATION AND HOME HEALTH CARE

To fully understand the role of the speech-language pathologist in home health care, the practitioner must understand the concept of rehabilitation in home health care in general. Of importance to the practicing clinician in home health care is the World Health Organization (1980) classification of impairment and disability. The classification defines impairment as an abnormality of structure or function at the organ level, disability as the functional consequences of an impairment, and handicap as the social consequences of the disability. Table 2–1 depicts this classification specific to speech-language pathology.

The goal of any rehabilitation discipline, including speech-language pathology, is to take a patient from dependence to functional independence. Dependence then can be defined as the amount of assistance queuing or prompting a patient may need in order to function, while functional independence can be defined as minimal or no assistance needed and timely and safe performance. Figure 2–1 is a model of the continuum of rehabilitation care.

Traditional models of care and home health were depicted as primarily transdisciplinary. Each discipline was responsible for its own evaluation and assessment, and coordination was not noticeable among the disciplines. However, during the mid- to late-1990s, there arose a great emphasis on interdisciplinary care. Today, there is even more emphasis on multiskilling of all disciplines treating people in the home. Figure 2–2 shows the traditional care model, and Figure 2–3 shows a conceptual model of interdisciplinary care. Speech-language pathologists must understand at what level their skills and treatment fit along the interdisciplinary continuum of care in relation to the patient's ability to carry out

Table 2–1 International Classification of Impairments, Disabilities, and Handicaps

	Impairment	Disability	Handicap
Definitions	Abnormality of structure or function at the organ level	Functional consequences of an impairment	Social consequences of an impairment or a disability
Examples	Speech, language, cognitive, hearing impairments	Communication problems in context of daily life activities	Isolation, joblessness, dependency, role changes
Outcome measures	Traditional instrumental and behavioral diagnostic measures	Functional status measures	Quality of life scales, handicap inventories, wellness measures

Source: Reprinted with permission from *International Classification of Impairments, Disabilities, and Handicaps*, © 1980, World Health Organization.

activities of daily living. The following are modalities of function for activities of daily living and their definitions:

- *Dressing* includes both dressing and undressing as necessary. Examples of indoor articles of clothing are appropriate underclothing, either a pullover or an open shirt properly fastened, pants or slacks (with or without belt), socks and shoes (fastened only as necessary), a housedress, and so forth. Also included is the ability to obtain necessary supplies to perform the activity.
- *Grooming* includes activities of hair care (combing, brushing); oral care, such as brushing teeth or dentures; makeup application; shaving; and body care (application of necessary lotions, powders, and deodorant). Also included is the ability to obtain necessary supplies to perform the activity.
- *Toileting* focuses on independence in management of elimination and includes the ability to get to and from the toilet, commode, or bedpan; appropriate transfers; and the ability to manage self-toileting and hygiene, including alternative methods such as a catheter or colostomy. Also included is the ability to obtain necessary supplies to perform the activity.

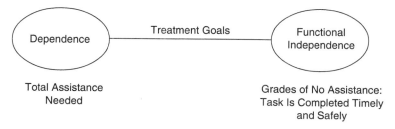

Figure 2–1 Continuum of Rehabilitation Care Model. *Source*: Copyright © 1998, Cecil G. Betros, Jr.

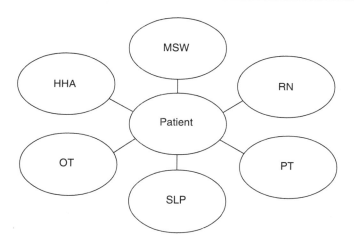

Figure 2–2 Traditional Care Model. *Source*: Copyright © 1998, Cecil G. Betros, Jr.

- *Washing and bathing* includes all aspects of bathing: mobility to get in and out of the tub or shower, with or without assistive devices, and washing and drying of the body, hair, face, and hands. A bed bath or sink bathing may be normal and adequate for some patients. Also included is the ability to obtain necessary supplies to perform the activity.
- *Feeding* focuses on independence and self-nourishment, whether through oral, enteral, or parenteral means. It includes the act of feeding as well as the setup of meals (if appropriate to the discharge situation), and also swallowing and pocketing with patients with dysphagia. However, food preparation is not included.

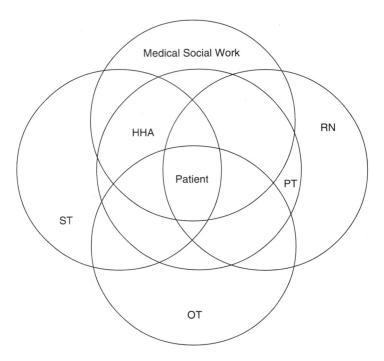

Figure 2–3 Interdisciplinary Care Model. *Source:* Copyright © 1998, Cecil G. Betros, Jr.

Speech-language pathologists must determine where speech, language, and/or cognition fit into assisting patients in becoming independent in their activities of daily living. In the activity of dressing, for example, the clinician must determine which language skills are necessary for the patient to be able to conduct the activity. First, the patient must be able to name the articles of clothing that he or she wants to use in dressing. The patient must also be able to gesture or demonstrate how the article of clothing is placed on the body. And, last but not least, the patient should be aware of the type of weather in order to put on the correct clothing. It is suggested that clinicians examine each activity of daily living and define for themselves how their treatment interventions and strategies cross interdisciplinary care. They will find that in home health care, the role of the speech-language pathologist is not an independent discipline in its entirety but a discipline that crosses all treating modalities.

DISTINGUISHING CHARACTERISTICS OF THE PROFESSION

Home health speech-language pathology refers to the practice of speech-language pathology applied to patients with speech, language, hearing, cognitive, and swallowing disorders in the patients' place of residence. Patients and their designated caregivers and/or significant others are the focus of home health speech-language pathology practice. The goal of care is to initiate, manage, and evaluate the resources needed to promote the patient's optimal level of communication, hearing, cognition, or swallowing. Speech-language pathology activities necessary to achieve this goal may include preventive, maintenance, and restorative programs to avoid potential deficits from developing.

The speech-language pathologist is a professional specialist in human communication, its normal development, and its disorders. As with other home care skilled specialty services, rigid postgraduate clinical training requirements and state licensure laws guarantee the quality of speech-language pathology services.

Home health speech-language pathology is a synthesis of the typically occurring practices of speech-language pathology and selected technical skills from other medical specialties. The speech-language cognitive or swallowing deficits of the patient determine the appropriate augmentation of other medical specialty skills with typically occurring speech-language pathology practice. As with community health nursing practices, speech-language pathology in home health includes care directed toward individual patients, families, and groups, with the predominant responsibility for care being to the population as a whole (Marrelli, 1994).

The practice of home health speech-language pathology is focused predominately on the care of the individual patient, in collaboration with the family, designated caregivers, and significant others. Home health speech-language pathology should foster the holistic management of personal health practices for the treatment of disease or disability. Practice activities center on treatment, care, and rehabilitation; assistance to families; direct treatment in the patient's residence; and coordination of community resources. Like nurses, home health speech-language pathologists acknowledge the biological, psychosocial, and environmental factors affecting their patients' health and illness protection, and they support a patient-focused speech-language pathology care plan addressing a comprehensive approach to goal achievement. During a patient's episode of care, technically precise speech-language pathology procedures may be instituted simultaneously with demands for teaching, counseling, care management, resource coordination, and evaluative data collection.

Technical and comprehensive clinical decision-making activities and collaboration in multidisciplinary practice further strengthen the autonomous and independent practice demands of home health speech-language pathology services. It is the speech-language pathology treatment process that is the essential vehicle through which the patient's goals are achieved.

Almost all speech-language pathology care is based on a complete physical, psychosocial, environmental, and speech-language pathology assessment. In the home setting, the influence of family dynamics and home environment on the physical, emotional, and communicative states of the patient are essential inclusions in the speech-language pathology plan of care. The patient, family, and caregivers are members of the health care team and will contribute to the speech-language pathology plan of care and goals. Because the speech-language pathologist is a guest in the home, the dynamics of the clinician-patient relationship are unique.

In addition, the patient's immediate access to other health care resources in the home is limited, so the speech-language pathologist's role as a multidisciplinary care coordinator is important in facilitating the goal of care (see Figure 2–4). This information exchange and advocacy process is used to encourage patients, families, and caregivers to plan for and think about additional services as their needs and resources dictate. Informing, supporting, and affirming patient and caregiver determinism is an important adjunct to achieving the speech-language pathology care plan and patient goals.

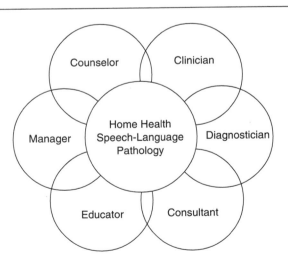

Figure 2–4 The Roles of Speech-Language Pathology in Home Health Care. *Source:* Copyright © 1998, Cecil G. Betros, Jr.

The Generalist Role

The professional home health speech-language pathologist practices at the generalist level in the patient's home, site of residence, or appropriate community site. The focus of the speech-language pathologist's practice includes the patient, family, and caregivers. Responsibilities of the speech-language pathologist in the role of generalist include teaching, performing speech-language pathology activities within the plan of care, managing resources needed to ensure enactment of the care plan, monitoring technical and instrumental care should the patient require it, communicating and collaborating with other disciplines and providers, and supervising ancillary personnel.

All professional clinicians practicing as home health speech-language pathologists should possess the basic knowledge and skills to carry out the following responsibilities:

- Perform holistic initial and periodic assessments of the patient, family, and caregiver resources to develop and support the speech-language pathology plan of care.
- Define and coordinate, in conjunction with other disciplines, the community resources necessary to support optimal patient outcomes.
- Use qualitative and quantitative analyses to evaluate patient responses to treatment and monitor the parameters of care according to the patient's plan of care.
- Educate and counsel patients, families, and caregivers to promote communicative independence and self-care activities.
- Initiate health promotion teaching to improve the quality of life, maintain health, and minimize disability.
- Implement the advocacy role through activities that inform, support, and affirm patient and family self-determination and functional independence.
- Promote continuity of care through discharge planning, case management, and advocacy.
- Apply the appropriate multidisciplinary knowledge and use of interdisciplinary care models to the practice of speech-language pathology.
- Recognize the biological, psychological, emotional, and social and environmental changes in patients, families, and caregivers based on an understanding of psychological, cultural, social, and spiritual functioning.
- Use practice standards and the appropriate state speech-language pathology acts to guide speech-language pathology evaluation and treatment procedures.
- Provide technical and instrumental care for the patient, as appropriate.

- Monitor and support family and caregiver participation in furthering the goals of patient care.

The Specialist Role

The speech-language pathologist working in the specialist role of home health care is usually one who possesses substantial clinical experience with individual patients, families, and groups; expertise in the process of caseload management and consultation; and proficiency in planning, implementing, and evaluating programs, resources, services, and research for health care delivery to patients with complex problems. In addition to these skills, the speech-language pathology specialist understands the federal guidelines in terms of service coverage and reimbursement issues.

One of the major areas of the specialist role for the speech-language pathologist is that of consultant. As a consultant, the speech-language pathologist should have knowledge and skills to carry out the following responsibilities:

- Provide consultation to staff clinicians who participate in the delivery of care.
- Design, monitor, evaluate, and consult with home health agencies in the continuous quality improvement process and risk management components of the clinical speech-language pathology program.
- Identify and design research projects based on data generated from the continuous quality improvement programs and clinical speech-language pathology observations.
- Serve as a resource to home health personnel in identification and evaluation of patients in need of speech rehabilitative care.
- Educate nurses, home health aides, other team members, and physicians regarding technical, cognitive, and clinical developments emerging for the home health patient in terms of communication, swallowing, hearing, and language.
- Perform direct patient care on a consultation basis and document for selected patients and caregivers who require the expertise of a specialist.
- Consult, manage, and evaluate the care delivered by caregivers to prevent the reoccurrence of communication deficits in complex cases.
- Monitor and evaluate trends and patterns of reimbursement for home health speech-language pathology.
- Consult and participate in developing and evaluating home health care agency policies and procedures to promote functional communication independence in homebound patients.
- Consult with staff and patients on ethical issues related to treatment and self-determinism.

Theoretical Foundations of Treatment

To understand the complexity of treating patients in their place of residence, one must have a good understanding of the traditional and theoretical foundations of communication disorders treatment. Traditionally, speech-language therapy has been just as behavioral as behavioral modification (the former derived pragmatically, the latter from operant learning principles). The same general therapeutic consideration underlies most of the methods for remediating speech. From assessment, speech-language pathologists determine the dimensions of the problems as precisely as possible. They make this determination by comparing what the patient does with what he or she should be able to do (Perkins, 1977). Holding this goal as the terminal behavior to be achieved, the clinician is ready to undertake therapy. The clinician must now find patient responses that can be systematically modified to the desired form: The more closely the patient approaches the terminal behavior, the less difficult the therapeutic task will be. In a word, the clinician must begin where the patient can perform without failure and, by careful selection of types and schedules of reinforcement, move step by step to the terminal goal. No step is taken until its success is ensured. At the first sign of failure, the clinician mounts a strategic retreat to a point at which successful performance can be reestablished (Perkins, 1977).

TRADITIONAL SERVICE SETTINGS

Speech-language pathologists offer a rather wide variety of services, depending upon the professional setting and the population served. Most clinicians provide diagnostic and treatment services, with fewer members of the profession offering consultation, training, and administration of clinical, academic, or governmental agencies. Still others are primarily engaged in research activities. Most speech-language pathologists are employed in public schools, community clinics, and hospitals. The remaining professionals are found in universities; local, state, and federal agencies; private practice; the armed forces; and private industry. The focus of this chapter is on home health care services directly related to serving older persons.

Because of the higher incidence of medical problems observed among older persons, hospitalization is certainly more probable in this group; therefore, a review of speech-language pathology services in the hospital setting would seem warranted. Stanbert (1977) examined such services in a comprehensive survey of hospitals. In the 717 responding hospitals, patients ranging from 45 to 64 years were the most frequently treated, and those over age 64 ranked second in frequency of treatment. The most frequently treated disorders, beginning with the most common, were as follows:

1. aphasia
2. apraxia
3. language disorders
4. articulation disorders
5. voice disorders
6. neurological disorders
7. cancer-related disorders
8. cleft palate
9. cerebral palsy

Neurologists constituted the most common referral source, followed in order by pediatricians, otolaryngologists, physiatrists, internists, general practitioners, psychiatrists, and orthopaedic surgeons.

The medical setting is the setting most like home health care. In most instances, speech-language pathology training programs do not offer extensive coursework or practice to prepare speech-language pathologists for any type of medical setting. Although some coursework may be offered in affiliated medical schools, the classroom training, in most cases, is not medically oriented and is taught outside the medical setting. The majority of practicum experiences are sponsored in university speech and hearing clinics, private rehabilitation centers, specialty schools such as those for patients with cerebral palsy or hearing impairments, and the public schools. Most of these settings are not directly affiliated with medical training programs and do not support inpatient hospital beds or home health care (Miller & Groher, 1990).

The speech-language pathologist is taught to diagnose and treat disorders of communication; however, many communication disorders tend to be secondary to a primary medical diagnosis, such as dysarthria that is secondary to the medical diagnosis of amyotrophic lateral sclerosis. For the speech-language pathologist in the typical medical setting, the role of diagnostician is diminished. Because most patients sent to the speech-language pathologist have a medical diagnosis, the referring physician may assume that the speech-language pathologist's diagnosis will be limited to whether or not the patient can benefit from communication intervention. Therefore, the physician typically does not expect any information that may be relevant to the primary medical diagnosis. This misguided assumption may lead physicians to limit the field of communication disorders more to aspects of rehabilitation than to the process of differential diagnosis. In fact, the speech-language pathologist must separate some communication disorders from others (e.g., speech from language) and distinguish among subtypes (e.g., Broca's from Wernicke's aphasia) by processes of differential diagnosis.

Speech-language pathologists in a typical medical setting will interact most often with the specialties of pediatrics, otolaryngology, neurology and neurosurgery, rehabilitation medicine, and nursing. Those who provide diagnostic guidance and treatment management of patients with dysphagia will spend additional time with dietitians, gastroenterologists, radiologists, and dentists. Other specialties, such as cardiology, pulmonology, and surgical specialties, will request speech-language pathology services on a more limited basis. To maintain successful interactions with all of these specialties, speech-language pathologists should know what types of patients should be referred to each of these services. This knowledge allows speech-language pathologists to be conversant regarding their findings from the perspective of communication specialists.

TYPICAL HOME CARE CASE TYPES

Rehabilitative speech-language pathology services can be offered for a wide variety of communication disorders. According to *Caring Magazine*, the following are typical home care communication disorders and their treatments ("In-Home Speech-Language," 1988):

- Hearing impairments are common among older persons. Communication disorders are typically found in the home health setting. The speech-language pathologist treats this disorder through hearing tests and aural rehabilitation to teach the patient how to speech read or lip-read. Auditory training is also used for hearing impairments.
- Swallowing disorders can be treated through oral muscle exercises, swallowing techniques, and appropriate diets that will ease the swallowing process.
- A loss of speech and language abilities can result from brain damage resulting from a stroke, mental retardation, a head injury, or a brain tumor. Speech-language pathology rehabilitative services in this situation are designed to help the patient relearn language, speech, and/or cognitive skills such as work recall, the ability to produce speech sounds, and/or the ability to write a check.
- A stroke or brain tumor may affect the speech muscles that are needed to produce a particular sound at the appropriate time, that is, dysarthria or apraxia of speech. A speech-language pathologist can help a patient with such a disability to increase the conscious control of the initiation, timing, and direction of speech motor movements.
- Inadequate respiratory volume and control often accompany neurological disorders. For such disorders, the speech-language pathologist assists the patient with developing proper control of the vocal and respiratory system for correct voice production.

- Voice loss is most frequently caused by the surgical removal of the vocal mechanism (laryngectomy) because of cancer. In such cases, the speech-language pathologist assists the patient with using other neck muscles for producing speech or electronic devices to create sound in the throat.

Regardless of the nature of the impairment, the patient is referred for speech-language pathology services only after an order from the patient's physician is obtained. The speech-language pathologist establishes the plan of care and the rehabilitation program in coordination with the patient's physician.

ASSESSMENT AND DEVELOPMENT OF INTERVENTION STRATEGIES

Rehabilitative management of communication disorders in the home is the responsibility of the speech-language pathologist, with the physician acting as a consultant for pre- and post-treatment examinations. Many communication disorders seen in the home result from cerebral malfunction and/or damage, dysfunction of the neurological integrity of the patient, or cancer, all of which may cause impaired communication, oral-facial muscle weakness or paresis, and swallowing disorders. These changes in the patient's communicative ability necessitate evaluative and therapeutic procedures provided by a speech-language pathologist, whose primary role is the diagnosis and rehabilitation of various communication disorders. Additionally, speech-language pathologists have the responsibility for referring patients to other specialists when necessary to supplement therapeutic management.

Assessment Methodologies

Initial Assessment

The speech-language pathologist's initial responsibility with the homebound patient is to identify specific (presumably aberrant) communication dysfunctions and associated abnormal behaviors. This task involves specific diagnostic testing and an initial interview to obtain case history information. Early in the diagnostic process, the speech-language pathologist ensures that the patient and family or significant others understand why the patient was referred for treatment and provides information about the patient's particular communication disorder. Often patients and their families have not fully understood explanations by the physician and need to be reassured that the condition is treatable. It is imperative, however, that the speech-language pathologist use terminology that is easily understood by the patient and family and encourage the patient to ask questions about his or her condition.

Case history information is an important aspect of the overall diagnostic process. The case history includes general identifying information about the patient and details about his or her family, schoolwork situation (if any), health, and premorbid communication habits. Information about the duration of the communication disorder is obtained, and an attempt must be made to date its origin and the circumstances that precipitated it. The patient's working environment should be considered with respect to the amount of communication necessary and the overall style of the patient's communication. For example, if the patient was a professor, and thus communication was a valuable part of his or her existence, then a stroke-causing aphasia could have a devastating effect on his or her emotional well-being. Domestic quarrels between husband and wife or arguments and disagreements with children can be significant information for the speech-language pathologist in developing an intervention plan. Consideration must be given to the patient's general health, especially if he or she is fatigued after treatment sessions, is lethargic, or is taking a significant amount of medications.

The diagnosis of communication disorders in the home should be related to the information from the case history, and factors contributing to the condition must be carefully observed and noted. These factors can be noted while one is taking the case history and during specific testing. It may also be useful to have the patient, family, or significant other describe the patient's communication abilities before the onset of the current problem, especially if certain distinctive patterns are apparent during evaluation that could not be considered to be directly related to the present communication dysfunction. Ideally, the speech-language pathologist must be able to identify the strengths and weaknesses of the patient's communication, including any imbalance in musculature and any problems with oral communication or understanding, by correlating the case history, specific tests, and the patient's current modes of communication. Current medications, family dynamics, and the history of the disease processes are ancillary to the total picture of the patient's current condition.

An hour is usually allowed for the initial speech/language/swallowing evaluation. Once all the necessary information is obtained, treatment is initiated immediately. All home care patients with communication dysfunction are given some direct suggestions for communication with family and significant others before the diagnostic session ends. These tips provide concrete evidence to the patient, family, and significant others that the interventions will be structured and that improvement is possible. Ideally, home care patients with communication disorders should be seen daily, but because of federal regulations, patients are usually seen two to three times weekly.

Assessment of the Environment

When treatment visits are made to the patient's home, the speech-language pathologist also must evaluate the home environment. Assessment of family support systems is important to communication rehabilitation in the home setting. In the patient's home, family or significant others are needed not only to provide physical and emotional support to the patient but also to serve as a vehicle to the communication process itself. Encouraging the patient to use shorter sentences, prompting the patient to speak louder, asking the patient to exaggerate the pronunciation of words, and giving feedback about the listener's ability to understand what the patient said are specific ways in which the family can contribute to the improvement of communication situations. Additionally, instruction of family support members in the implementation of the patient's maintenance programs is important to the patient's treatment progress.

Intervention Strategies

In speech/language/swallowing rehabilitation for the homebound patient, early emphasis is placed on establishing some mode of communication for the patient. Exercises in word recall, oral-motor exercises to strengthen the oral-facial muscles, and listening exercises, in most cases, are started at once to facilitate the foundation of good oral communication.

Treatment follows a logical plan, which encompasses the introduction of careful facilitating exercises, usually progressing from improving general communication skills to more specific procedures directed at the patient's communication dysfunction. Exercises practiced in the home are written in a notebook and recorded on a sheet to ensure that the patient does not forget instructions or waste time between treatment sessions in practicing exercises incorrectly, or not at all. Most patients, families, and significant others, however, are conscientious about practice, especially if they are motivated to have the patient communicate, go back to work, or function in activities of daily living. The best exercises are those that the patient can consciously apply while speaking in everyday situations.

SPECIAL SKILLS NEEDED BY THE SPEECH-LANGUAGE PATHOLOGIST

Note: Although there are no data to support the description in this section of the special skills needed by speech-language pathologists, experience has shown that these skills are necessary and that they help to establish the speech-language pathologist as part of the medical team.

Working in home health care requires, to some extent, a sophisticated level of life experiences. Home care is not the place for immature clinicians who are unsure of themselves. Clinicians must remember that they treat the patient in his or her home, or turf, and they therefore must be respectful of the patient's everyday routine and living environment. The clinician is the guest. Clinicians working in other clinical environments that are more traditional in nature (e.g., speech and hearing centers, rehabilitation agencies, and hospitals) have medical personnel readily available for emergencies. The home health speech-language pathologist must rely on his or her own training, intuition, and initiative to intervene with medical problems that might arise.

Traditional speech-language pathology "on the job training" is only part of the education of the home health speech-language pathologist, who must also be knowledgeable in basic medical emergency techniques. In addition, nursing and other health care professionals are not immediately available to assist the speech-language pathologist with medical signs and symptoms. For example, speech-language pathologists must be able to take a temperature, pulse, and respiration. They do not interpret this information but must communicate it to the correct medical personnel. For example, a patient at home may have a swallowing dysfunction, causing the patient to aspirate foods and/or liquids. If that patient is spiking a temperature, material could have been aspirated into the lungs, which could then lead to pneumonia. For speech-language pathologists to assist with medical decisions about the patient's need for medication or hospitalization, it is critical that they report vital signs so that the appropriate interventions can take place. The vast majority of patients seen in the home for speech-language pathology are those who have had a cerebrovascular accident (CVA) or some other disorder that has decreased the integrity of the cerebrovascular and/or neurological systems. In addition, some patients have had transient ischemic attacks (TIAs), in which the blood flow to the brain is temporarily stopped or decreased. In these cases, one can see fluctuations in responses, level of alertness, and blood pressure. The clinician's ability to take blood pressure in this instance is critical to the team, as this information is needed to prevent further cerebrovascular damage or another stroke.

Infection control has become a primary concern of health care workers today. Stringent federal guidelines require strict precautionary measures for bloodborne pathogens such as hepatitis B and other infectious diseases. No instrument can be taken from one patient's house to another without proper infection control techniques. For example, clinicians must wash their hands upon entering a patient's home and after completion of the clinical session. Any treatment materials used must be on plain plastic while in use. In addition, a large majority of patients are insulin-dependent diabetic persons. Most are receiving one or more insulin injections per day. Clinicians are always cautioned regarding any type of syringes found in the home. Federal guidelines also require gloves and masks any time a clinician is working in or around an area where body fluids could be exchanged.

Federal guidelines require health care providers to attend at least one inservice per year on bloodborne pathogens.

It is recommended that clinicians also have the following competencies:

- general knowledge of pharmacology and medicine interactions
- ability to recognize signs of patient distress
- ability to take a temperature, pulse, and respiration
- knowledge of disease processes and their effects on communication
- dysphagia training, especially in bedside techniques
- training in cervical auscultation, a technique whereby a stethoscope is placed on the neck near the area of the laryngeal mechanism to listen for abnormal swallowing sounds
- basic counseling techniques

In addition, the Health Care Financing Administration and the Joint Commission on Accreditation of Healthcare Organizations mandate the following for speech-language pathologists:

- Each clinician must be certified in cardiopulmonary resuscitation (CPR).
- Each clinician must be educated regarding advance directives.
- Each clinician must understand what safety issues exist in the home.
- Each clinician must be knowledgeable in infection control.

Contributions to Interdisciplinary Teams

Speech-language pathologists often participate in monthly meetings where health care professionals come together to discuss the patient's care from the viewpoints of the represented disciplines. In particular, the patient's current medical status and prognosis are presented from each discipline's standpoint, together with recommendations for treatment and any report on the effects of treatment already completed.

These meetings help to integrate the services of each discipline into a harmonious style, in accordance with the home health agency's policies and procedures. Discussions revolve around problematic cases, patients who have received services for more than 60 days, and those cases involving multiple disciplines. Documentation is then entered into the corresponding patient record. The home care department also establishes a designated time when the therapists, social workers, and home health aide agency can contact the nurse and patient care manager to discuss case management issues that cannot wait until the team meeting.

Because the care of the patient by many other disciplines depends largely on the patient's ability to understand and communicate, speech-language pathologists have an integral role in regard to interdisciplinary teams. For example, a nurse may be teaching a patient about his or her medicines, what they are and when to take them. If the patient has comprehension problems, the nurse will not be able to complete the education. In addition, a vast majority of physical therapy exercises for homebound patients require sequencing of motor acts. If a patient is unable to sequence items or understand verbal instructions, the physical therapist will be unable to carry out the exercise program. Speech-language pathologists therefore must be able to establish an appropriate communication system between the nurse and other therapists and the patient and family. Methods might include teaching signs, using communication boards, or even working on interpersonal skills training.

Dysphagia Management

In the past 15 years, speech-language pathology in the management of patients with dysphagia has been on the rise. Unlike acute care settings, the home care environment can present many interesting modifications of the typical management of dysphagia. The most frequently occurring modification of typical dysphagia treatment in the home is usually the lack of medical information. Most often, the patient has not had a modified barium swallow, or the report sent to the agency is not current. Thus, the home health speech-language pathologist must become skilled in the bedside evaluation of dysphagia. In addition, patient and family compliance issues in regard to swallowing safety become of primary concern. It is sometimes difficult for them to prepare pureed food or an altered diet for the patient. A large majority of dysphagia treatment involves compliance with swallowing safety issues.

At times, there has been some controversy over the differing roles of the speech-language pathologist and the occupational therapist in regard to who is responsible for the patient with swallowing difficulty. In the 90 agencies that work with Communication Concepts and Consulting, Inc., the responsibility for management of patients with dysphagia rests with the speech-language pathologist. The occupational therapist is responsible for the motor act of getting food into the patient's mouth, but it is the responsibility of the speech pathologist to get the bolus into the stomach once it enters the mouth.

RURAL HOME HEALTH

According to criteria set by the U.S. Census Bureau, a standard metropolitan statistical area (SMSA) is defined as one with a population of 100,000 or more. The U.S. Bureau of the Census (1980) defines a rural area as any nonmetropolitan aggregate with less than 2,500 people residing in open country. "Open country" is considered to be an area with a population density of one to six persons per square mile. By this definition, about 27 percent of the U.S. population is rural.

Rural home health care can present some precarious situations for the home health speech-language pathologist. Patients often are seen in subnormal housing without flooring or indoor plumbing. Lighting can also be an obstacle with the rural population, since occasionally a household has no electricity. In addition, during the summer and winter months, proper cooling and heating can be an issue for not only the clinician but also the family. For example, the father of one rural Alabama family was in an urban rehabilitation hospital. Upon discharge from the rehab hospital, the patient went home, where his daughter was to care for him. After approximately one month, the daughter decided to make living quarters for her father. When the clinician arrived, the patient was living in a home made of cardboard with no facilities.

Driving hazards in rural areas can also become obstacles to treatment. Many rural residents live on dirt roads or on routes. Directions to the patient's home can be difficult to understand, since the environment, rather than road signs, is sometimes used as a guide. In addition, heavy rains can prevent the clinician from making a visit to the patient who lives on a dirt road.

CONCLUSION

The speech-language pathologist working in the home care arena has an arduous task but an exciting responsibility. The qualitative skills of speech-language pathologists working in home care, combined with proper planning and patience, can enable home care patients with communication disorders to bridge the communication gap and make great strides toward increasing their ability to interact with others.

REFERENCES

In-home speech-language pathology services. (1988). *Caring Magazine, 19,* 16–17.

Marrelli, T.M. (1994). *Handbook of home health standards and documentation guidelines for reimbursement.* St. Louis, MO: CV Mosby.

Miller, R.M., & Groher, M.E. (1990). *Medical speech pathology.* Rockville, MD: Aspen Publishers.

Perkins, W.H. (1977). *Speech pathology: An applied behavioral science.* St. Louis, MO: CV Mosby.

Stanbert, T.E. (1977). A national study of United States hospital speech pathology services (Report No. 1). *ASHA, 19,* 160–163.

U.S. Bureau of the Census. (1980). *Characteristics of rural and farm-related population* (Publication No. PC 80-2.9). Washington, DC: Author.

World Health Organization. (1980). *International classification of impairments, disabilities, and handicaps.* Geneva, Switzerland: Author.

SUGGESTED READING

Paden, E.P. (1970). *A history of the American Speech and Hearing Association, 1925–1958.* Washington, DC: American Speech and Hearing Association.

Van Riper, C. (1971). *Speech correction: Principles and methods.* Englewood Cliffs, NJ: Prentice Hall.

PART II

Steps in the Assessment Process

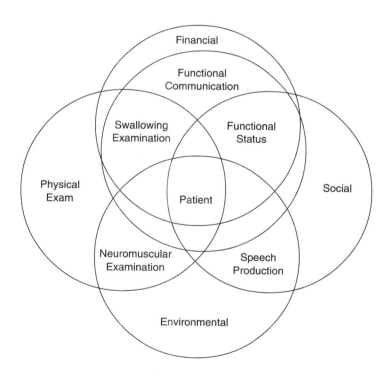

CHAPTER 3

The Referral and Home Visit Process

INTRODUCTION

A referral is the avenue of communication through which cases are directed to a service provider, for example, a home health care agency. This chapter presents an overview of case management from initial source referral through the evaluation of care using what might be called the *speech-language pathology process*. Unique strategies for increasing referrals to speech-language pathology in home health care are also discussed.

THE REFERRAL PROCESS

Each agency has specific procedures and forms for handling referrals. Although procedures may vary from agency to agency, many are common to most areas of home health practice (Figure 3–1). Speech-language pathologists should become familiar with the procedures implemented by each agency for which they work. They will then be able to assess patients more effectively and in a more timely and appropriate manner.

After receiving a referral, but before scheduling the initial visit, the speech-language pathologist should confer with the case manager, team leader, or other team members to ensure the coordination of services. Communication helps to maximize care and clearly delineate the role of each team member. The speech-language pathologist should then contact the patient and his or her family or caregiver to make an appointment for the initial visit.

The routing of a referral varies from agency to agency also, so policy on the timeliness of the initial visit may differ. However, most agencies require an admission to be completed within 48 to 72 hours for rehabilitation services. When the initial visit has been completed, the speech-language pathologist completes a

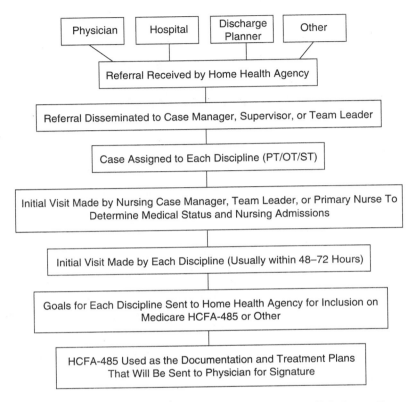

Figure 3–1 The Referral Process. *Source:* Copyright © 1998, Cecil G. Betros, Jr.

summary of the evaluation, identifying the patient's problems and needs, and establishes a plan of care. For Medicare, this information must be recorded on a specific form (HCFA-485, see service codes for this form in Appendix C) and is submitted to the referring physician for a signature. The form should be completed according to the policies and procedures of the individual agency and its fiscal intermediary. For reimbursement sources other than Medicare, many agencies have developed their own baseline data forms. Some agencies have separate physician order forms for each discipline, while others use the integrated form.

Sources of Referrals to Speech-Language Pathology

Referrals for home health care come from a variety of sources. They may originate from acute care settings, physicians, registered nurses, physical therapists, patients themselves, occupational therapists, social workers, families, or community advocates. Referrals to a home health care agency may also come from other agencies providing patient care such as rehab centers, extended care facilities, nursing homes, community health facilities, clinics, and centers for individuals who are disabled. In addition, agencies in another geographic area may refer patients. For example, a home care patient moves to another state, but the patient requires further therapy and will still be homebound after relocating. The agency that previously treated the patient refers him or her to a home health care agency in the new place of residence, and a physician is contacted there to assume responsibility for prescribing and signing orders for continued home health services.

Typically, hospitals and skilled nursing facilities have discharge planners or social service departments that plan for a patient's return home. Also, some home health care agencies hire individuals, often nurses or social workers, to go into hospitals or skilled facilities to serve as discharge planners and perform case findings for the agencies' area. Before a patient leaves an institution, a discharge planner not only refers the patient to an appropriate agency but also helps to organize the home health care program. This process may include assessing the need for durable medical equipment, skilled nursing care, home health aide services, and appropriate rehabilitation services. Ideally, the discharge planner would confer with the physician, floor nurses, rehab staff, and patient's family before arranging for provision of any services or equipment. It must be noted, however, that this system is not typical.

Referral Assignment

In large home health care agencies, 500 referrals a month are usually received by an intake coordinator, who is often a nurse or may be a qualified secretary, if state regulations permit. This person gives copies of the referral to the case manager, supervisor, or team leader. When the referral includes orders for speech-language pathology services, the case manager, supervisor, or team leader assigns the case to an appropriate speech-language pathologist or speech-language pathology group.

In small agencies, a nurse may receive the referral and forward it directly to the professional or professionals who will provide the requested services. Speech-language pathologists may receive the referral by phone, mail, or (more typically) fax, and on occasion they may be expected to pick up the information at the agency.

Referral Information

Typically, a referral to speech-language pathology in a home health care agency is received from one of two sources. The first is the original source that referred the patient to home health care to initiate services. For example, a discharge planner in a hospital may refer the patient to a home health care agency and indicate what services are generally needed or should be ordered. In this case, the agency-level referral form (Exhibit 3–1) is the most typical document used to initiate speech-language pathology services. The request for speech-language pathology services is generally a broad one with unspecific goals and orders.

The second most common avenue for a referral to speech-language pathology and home health care comes from a home health care team member who has already been seeing the patient and has identified a need for speech-language pathology services. In the latter case, it is a good idea for speech-language pathologists to develop a referral form specific to their program. The purpose of such a form is to cue other team members to the unique contributions that speech-language pathology can offer and encourage questions about specific concerns that can be addressed by the speech-language pathologist. No matter what forms are used by the agency or developed by the speech-language pathologist, certain elements should be included (see Exhibit 3–2).

Some agencies prefer referral forms that are used to initiate multiple services, but the information provided is general and offers limited information to the providers of the service. Requests for services may also be very vague and incomplete. Ideally, cues are included on the form to encourage more specific orders other than "evaluate and treat as needed."

After the team member who opens the case makes the initial evaluation visit, he or she may determine the need for further treatment or service. At this time, an ancillary referral form can be used that supplements the original with orders for additional treatment or services. This form may be written following a phone call to the physician for oral orders and then sent to the physician for signature.

Increasing Referrals

Strategies for increasing referrals to speech-language pathology in home care include the following:

- When time permits, make home visits with nurses and nurses' aides.
- Provide inservice training to staff, nurses, and intake coordinators in brief presentations at staff meetings.
- Have lunch with marketing, public relations, and community relations staff and intake coordinators.
- Educate the agency staff network by participating in competency training sessions, student orientations, and care planning meetings.
- Review intake referrals and participate in agency-required clinical records review activities to find potential patients. Look for reports of dependence in

Exhibit 3–1 Generic Home Health Referral Form

MR #: _____   NURSING TEAM: _____

Admission #: _____   SOC: _____

Name: _____ DOB: _____ Race: _____

Street Address: _____ Phone: _____

Second Street Address: _____ Religion: _____

City, State, ZIP: _____ Sex: ____ Marital Status: _____

Directions to Address: _____
_____
_____
_____

Service Location: _____ Primary Caregiver: _____
Living Arrangements: _____ Emergency Contact Person: _____
   ❑ Diagnosis: _____ ICDA CODE: _____
   ❑ Diagnosis: _____ ICDA CODE: _____
   ❑ Diagnosis: _____ ICDA CODE: _____

Primary Physician: _____ Type: _____
UPIW #: _____ OFFICE NAME: _____

Street Address: _____
City, State, ZIP: _____
Phone: _____ Fax: _____

NOTIFICATION:
   ❑ Skilled nursing
   ❑ Physical therapy
   ❑ Speech-language pathology
   ❑ Occupational therapy
   ❑ Medical social work
   ❑ Home health aide

                 Admitted by: _____

Source: Copyright © 1998, Cecil G. Betros, Jr.

Exhibit 3–2 Guidelines: Elements To Include in Forms

The Patient
- The patient's name, address, telephone number, and date of birth
- How to contact the patient if there is no phone (e.g., through a relative or a neighbor or by going directly to the patient's home)
- Who to contact if the patient is unable to reach or speak on a telephone or does not speak English
- The patient's primary language and availability of interpreter
- Family members' names, addresses, and telephone numbers
- Instructions for entry (e.g., "Use side door" or "Call 15 minutes before the visit so that the door may be opened")
- Directions to the patient's home

Referring Physician
- The referring physician, or patient's physician, if referral is from another source
- Physician's name, address, and telephone number
- Physician's ID number

Primary Diagnosis
- Diagnosis for which agency care is requested
- Date of onset
- Dates of hospital stays if the patient has been admitted for treatment

Secondary Diagnosis
- Other medical and physical problems, with dates of onset, that affect the patient's ability to function
- Validation of the need for service at home
- Confirmation of the patient's homebound status

Medications
- Medications the patient is taking, including doses and frequency
- Special diets that the patient must follow
- Any allergies the patient has
- Name and telephone number of the patient's pharmacy

Payment Source
- Patient care reimbursement source (Medicare, Medicaid, major medical coverage, private insurance, United Way, etc.)
- Visit limits imposed by the third-party payer, if any

continues

Exhibit 3–2 continued

Date for Start of Service
• Date referral source wants each specific service to begin
(A nursing visit and an evaluation of the need for a home health aide may be necessary before, at the time of, or after the patient's return home.)

Services, Frequency of Visits, and Duration
• Services to be provided to the patient, how often, and for how long
(In some agencies, therapy and intervention decisions are left to the judgment of the nurse and the therapist. Treatment is often determined by the nurse or the therapist after the evaluation visit.)

Contraindications or Precautions to Treatment
• Cardiac or respiratory problems
• Seizures
• Intermittent stroke
• Transient ischemic attacks

Information about the Referral Source
• Person making the referral
• Source of referral
• Relationship of referring individual to the patient
• Condition on which referral source is judging the patient's needs for home health care
• Patient's level of function before onset of the illness or disability
• Homebound status, that is, whether the patient is able to leave the house with ease or needs maximum assistance

The Care Environment
• Who is in the home to assist the patient?
• Does the patient live alone?
• Does the patient have a home health aide?
• Who are the patient's significant others?

Source: Copyright © 1998, Cecil G. Betros, Jr.

communication, poor understanding, inability to follow directions, and poor cognitive skills.
• Network with hospital-based speech-language pathologists regarding their patients who are ready for discharge. A speech-language pathologist can provide a continuation of the acute care patient care plan to assess the patient for functional abilities in communication.

- Become a member of the agency's professional advisory board. It is important for the speech-language pathologist to provide at least an annual inservice to the advisory board on communication disorders found in the home.
- Participate in the agency's team meetings and/or utilization review committee meetings, which are great forums for case finding. Listen to cases presented by other disciplines in order to identify where the speech-language pathologist could have played a role in patient care.

CONDUCTING A HOME VISIT

After the referral has been received and processed, the next step in the speech-language pathology process is the home visit process, which consists of assessment, diagnosis and planning, intervention, and evaluation.

Assessment

Visit Preparation

Speech-language pathologists should prepare for the home visit by reviewing the referral form and any other pertinent information that is available concerning the patient. They may need to call the nurse, physician, or other rehabilitation specialists to get information. The first home visit provides the speech-language pathologist with the opportunity to establish a trust relationship with the patient and family and to establish credibility as a resource for health information in a nonthreatening environment.

The Referral. The referral is a formal request for a speech-language pathology visit. Referrals to the home health agency come from a variety of sources, including acute care hospitals, rehabilitation hospitals, clinics, health care providers, individuals, and families. In the Birmingham, Alabama, area, there are two large rehabilitation hospitals. Typically, stroke patients are soon admitted to these facilities postonset from the acute care hospital setting. Therefore, the majority of patients seen in this area would come from the rehabilitation hospitals.

Home health referrals are requested to provide short-term, intermittent skilled services and rehabilitation to patients and their families. For example, a patient who has had a stroke requires skilled nursing assessments, physical therapy for gait training, speech therapy for improvement of a speech deficit, and occupational therapy for retraining in activities of daily living such as bathing and cooking.

Review of the referral form before the first visit gives the speech-language pathologist basic information about the patient such as name, age, diagnosis, health status, address, telephone number, insurance coverage (if any), reason for referral, and source of the referral.

Additional information provided in the home health referral includes current patient medications, prescribed diet, other disciplines involved in the care of the patient, physician orders, and/or goal of care. This information is important because it gives the speech-language pathologist a picture of the patient.

Initial Telephone Contact. The patient and family are contacted by the speech-language pathologist and informed of the referral for service. The first telephone contact with the patient or family consists of an exchange of essential information, including an introduction and an explanation of the purpose of the visit by the speech-language pathologist. After this initial information is exchanged, the patient is informed of the speech-language pathologist's desire to make the initial visit, permission is received from the patient and/or family, and a mutually acceptable time is set for the visit. Because the speech-language pathologist is considered a guest in the patient's home, it is important that the patient and/or family understand and agree to the visit. The speech-language pathologist verifies the patient's address and asks for specific directions to the patient's home.

Not all patients have a telephone. If this is the case, the speech-language pathologist contacts the home health agency for a telephone number where messages can be left. If the patient does not have a telephone, the speech-language pathologist may choose to make a drop-in visit. This type of visit consists of an unannounced visit to the patient's home during which the speech-language pathologist explains the purpose of the referral, receives the patient's permission for the visit, and sets up a time for a future visit with the patient.

If the patient and/or family are not at home for the drop-in visit, the speech-language pathologist leaves an official agency care message and a brief note asking the patient and/or family to contact the home health agency to schedule the visit (Exhibit 3–3). The speech-language pathologist informs the home health agency that the visit was attempted but the patient was unavailable for contact. The clinician's primary responsibility when unsuccessful in locating the patient is to keep the home health agency, physician, or referring agency informed of the speech-language pathologist's efforts to establish contact with the patient and family.

Environmental Assessment

An environmental assessment begins as the speech-language pathologist leaves the office en route to the patient's home. Keating and Kelman (1988) suggest that clinicians use these questions to guide their assessment:

- How does the patient's neighborhood compare with other neighborhoods in the area?
- Are there adequate shopping facilities, such as grocery stores, close to the patient's home?

Exhibit 3–3 Official Agency Care Message

SORRY I MISSED YOU

YOUR SPEECH-LANGUAGE PATHOLOGIST WAS HERE

DATE/DAY AND TIME

I'LL PLAN TO COME BACK

DATE/DAY AND TIME

IF YOU CANNOT SEE ME THEN, PLEASE CALL MY OFFICE AT

THANKS!

The speech-language pathologist should also make note of the patient's home, that is, whether the patient lives in a single-family home, a single room in a home or hotel, an apartment, or a shared apartment or house. Specific assessments include the following:

- Is the patient's residence easily accessible by the patient, given the patient's age and functional ability?
- Are facilities for persons with disabilities available as necessary?
- Is the residence in an area with high rates of drug abuse or crime?
- Does the patient live alone?
- Does the patient have food in the home?
- Are there rodents, cockroaches, or other potential vectors of disease present in the patient's home?
- Does the patient's home have hot running water, heat, sanitation facilities, and adequate ventilation?
- Is the patient's residence safe relative to the patient's physical status, or is the home cluttered with debris and furniture?

The speech-language pathologist who works in home health care is aware of the environment and surroundings when making a home visit. On occasion, the speech-language pathologist may not feel safe entering the patient's home environment. For example, a speech-language pathologist may arrive at a home and discover that the patient lives in a drug house where drugs are being openly sold. In this situation, the speech-language pathologist should not enter the home but may call the patient and make arrangements to meet the patient at another location, if possible. No speech-language pathologist is expected to disregard personal safety in an effort to make a home visit.

Physical Assessment

During the first home visit, the type of patient assessment will vary depending on the type of communication disorder exhibited by the patient. The speech-language pathologist assesses the patient's knowledge of the patient's health status and communication efforts. The speech-language pathologist identifies knowledge deficits and uses this information in development of a plan of care.

Subjective information is obtained from the patient and the patient's family and includes the patient's perception of the situation and what the patient identifies as communication problems. The speech-language pathologist assesses whether the patient is isolated physically or socially from others and whether the patient is a member of a close-knit, nurturing, supportive family or kinship network. The amount of support that the patient perceives to be available may or may not be accurate, so the speech-language pathologist asks several questions about the patient's family, friends, and daily routine to assess the patient's level of social support.

The speech-language pathologist assesses the patient's communication skills and performs a speech/language/swallowing assessment, which includes a review of all systems that affect the patient's communication abilities, with an emphasis on the area affected by the patient's presenting condition. The speech-language pathologist obtains objective data through the use of essential diagnostic testing and clinical observation. The speech/language/swallowing assessment also includes information regarding the patient's functional communication status (e.g., how the patient currently communicates with family and friends). Assessment of the functional communication status is important for Medicare reimbursement and for the development of an individualized speech-language pathology care plan.

This assessment includes information regarding the patient's ability to make his or her wants and needs understood by family members, to perform activities of daily living independently, and to use assistive devices. Specific functional limitations, such as shortness of breath or muscle weakness, are assessed at this time. Information obtained during the assessment phase is used to identify the speech-language pathologist's diagnoses and to develop a plan of care.

Diagnosis and Planning

Develop a Plan for the Patient and Family

After the assessment phase of the home visit, the speech-language pathologist develops a plan of care for the patient and the family. This plan is developed with the patient and family. Often, the speech-language pathologist will develop a contract with the patient that delineates the role of the speech-language pathologist regarding the patient's communication and the role of the patient and the patient's family regarding exercises and carryover activities.

The goal of the home visit for the speech-language pathologist is to involve the patient in taking an active role in communication. It is important to ensure that the patient does not become dependent on the speech-language pathologist's interventions, because the clinician's involvement is short term.

Outline the Patient and Family Roles

Written contracts are helpful for both the speech-language pathologist and the patient because contracts clearly delineate both individuals' roles in implementation of the plan (Spradley, 1990). The written contract is used as a reference regarding the roles. The contract can be modified by mutual agreement of the patient and speech-language pathologist.

Intervention

Implementation of the care plan begins during the first home visit. The speech-language pathologist begins to provide the patient and family with information concerning the patient's communication status and the availability and accessibility of community resources and also provides skilled speech-language pathology care. At the end of the initial home visit, the speech-language pathologist discusses with the patient and family the need for additional home visits to treat the communication disorder. The speech-language pathologist discusses the goals of treatment and what to expect on the next visit. The patient and family are informed about any information or skills the speech-language pathologist will provide during the course of treatment, and the days or dates that treatment will take place are determined.

The speech-language pathologist terminates the first visit when the assessment is completed and a plan of care is established with the patient and family. The average first visit should not be longer than one hour. Much information is provided to the patient and family during that hour, and much information is collected by the speech-language pathologist. Most patients are tired by the end of a one-hour visit and often cannot retain any additional information provided by the speech-language pathologist. It is preferable to set a date for subsequent home visits to reinforce information provided and to work progressively toward achieving goals.

Evaluation

Evaluation of Progress toward Goals

The evaluation process is continuous and allows the speech-language pathologist to determine the achievement of or progress toward the goals identified for the patient and family. Input from the patient and family are critical to determine whether the goals established are realistic and achievable for the patient.

Modification of the Plan as Needed

The evaluation process also allows the speech-language pathologist and patient or family to discuss what is working well and where modifications are needed in the plan of care. Evaluation occurs through open communication between the speech-language pathologist and the patient and family, with the speech-language pathologist asking questions about specific parts of the care plan and testing the patient's communication in functional activities as outlined in the plan of care.

When Goals Have Been Achieved

The overall purpose of speech-language pathology home visits is to assist the patient and family by providing the information and speech-language pathology interventions necessary for the patient to function successfully on an independent basis. When the care plan goals are achieved, the speech-language pathologist is no longer needed by the patient. Discharge planning begins approximately upon admission, and the patient and family have input in the month prior to actual discharge, which gives them an opportunity to function without a skilled service involved.

CONCLUSION

The referral is the basis for the caseload of the speech-language pathologist providing home health care. It is evident that there are many strategies for finding cases. Referral information includes many elements that will guide the speech-language pathologist in designing meaningful treatment programs. Finally, the process of conducting a home visit must be organized and well planned. The clinician must obtain all pertinent data to facilitate the proper assessments and intervention strategies.

REFERENCES

Keating, S.B., & Kelman, G.B. (1988). *Home health care nursing.* Philadelphia: J.B. Lippincott Co.

Spradley, B.W. (1990). *Community health nursing concepts and practice* (3rd ed.). Boston: Little, Brown and Company.

SUGGESTED READING

The American Occupational Therapy Association, Inc. (1995). *Guidelines for occupational therapy practice in home health.* Bethesda, MD: Author.

Home Health Agency Assembly in New Jersey. (1985). *Guidelines for utilization of specialized rehabilitation services in home health agency* (Rev. ed.). Princeton, NJ: Author.

Jansak, J. (1990). Medicare part A provider costs: Are they allowable? *Home Health Line, 15,* 97–108.

CHAPTER **4**

Assessment Considerations in Home Health Care

INTRODUCTION

Speech-language pathology services provided in the home environment are a very effective means of maximizing a patient's functional communicative independence. Home-based speech, language, swallowing, and cognitive therapy is a natural extension of the profession's multifaceted and versatile techniques and enables a patient to become more communicative in the home environment. This chapter discusses unique home health clinical considerations when one is working with patients who have communication/swallowing/cognitive disorders.

GENERAL CONSIDERATIONS

Speech/language/swallowing evaluations in the home differ considerably from those encountered in a clinic or hospital. A wide variety of factors cannot be controlled, although the clinician has to deal with them. Some of the factors might include the environmental setting, ethnic diversity, limited or no work space, and the presence of family members during the evaluation. Noise is usually a big factor in working with patients in their home: Television, telephones ringing, and just daily outside noises can be a distraction for both the patient and the clinician.

Time allotment for an evaluation also varies from the traditional setting. Patients typically seen in the home are not able to withstand several hours of diagnostic testing. Also, third-party payers usually do not reimburse for more than 60 minutes in the home, so the clinician must have expert diagnostic abilities.

Adaptation of diagnostic tests is a major consideration in home evaluation. A typical aphasia test battery, for example, is usually standardized in hospitals or in outpatient settings. Therefore, when a clinician attempts to administer the same test in the home, the test's validity in the home environment might differ, and this should be stated in the evaluation report.

Clinicians also must be aware of infection control standards required in the home health environment and the proper procedures to be taken to ensure the protection of patients and themselves. Appendix 4–A is a summary of the principles of universal precautions and body substance isolation of the Occupational Safety and Health Administration's (OSHA's) bloodborne pathogen standards.

ASSESSMENT CONSIDERATIONS

Safety

A fundamental role of the speech-language pathologist in the home is to teach functional communication and safety. In the home care setting, communication safety needs might include functional communication, emergency response mechanisms, and home safety management procedures such as swallowing safety and cognitive issues. Table 4–1 illustrates a few guidelines for these criteria in the home.

Table 4–1 Communication Safety in the Home

Evaluation Areas	Treatment Strategies
Functional communication: Dialing a telephone	Preprogrammed phone Autodial phone for emergencies Phone accessible in all rooms Patient knowledge of how and when to dial 911
Emergency communication	Portable phone to carry around to each room Push-button medical alert system such as Life-Line to alert hospital or ambulance
Inability to speak	Use of telecommunications device for the deaf (TDD) Use of minimal speech to make medical needs known Use of augmentative communication system
Swallowing	Heimlich maneuver for choking Cardiopulmonary resuscitation (CPR) Aspiration emergency techniques

Source: Copyright © 1998, Cecil G. Betros, Jr.

Patient safety also includes signs of negligence or abuse. The acuity levels of patients seen in the home are much higher than those of 10 years ago. And this leads to high levels of caregiver stress, which can provoke behaviors that are consistent with negligence and/or abuse. Sometimes these behaviors are subtle and must be pursued to determine whether the patient has indeed been mistreated physically and/or emotionally. The clinician is bound by law to report any suspicions of mistreatment to the home health agency for follow-up.

Speech Production and Intelligibility

Patients' ability to make their basic wants and medical needs known and understood has a profound impact on environmental safety and therefore should be a high priority in the initial evaluation, treatment, and family education. Table 4–2 contains some suggested areas of speech intelligibility assessment for the clinician to consider. The clinician must assess the patient's ability to communicate basic wants and medical needs, such as calling for help, getting needed medication, and so forth. In home health, speech production and intelligibility are often evaluated within the context of functional communication skills rather than word- or phoneme-specific considerations. The patient's ability to speak clearly is usually observed during the initial visit as the patient talks during everyday communication activities.

Naturally, a full neuromuscular evaluation of the speech mechanism also includes lateral and bilateral integration elements and an evaluation of praxis, visual-motor integration, and oral-motor control. A further delineation of sen-

---

Table 4–2 Speech Intelligibility

Evaluation Areas	*Assessment Strategies*
Functional speech	Observe patient speaking to various people if the opportunity exists. Assess how well the patient gets the message across to the listener. Check for cueing and prompting.
Speech interchange	Listen for consistency in speech production and intelligibility.
Neuromuscular coordination	Observe neuromuscular coordination of the oral-facial muscles during connected speech.

Source: Copyright © 1997, Cecil G. Betros, Jr.

sorimotor areas addresses sensory awareness and processing areas. In addition, the clinician should include a neuromusculoskeletal evaluation of the oral-facial swallowing structures, which should include range of motion, strength, endurance, reflexes, postural control, and alignment measurements to help complete the home health clinician's understanding of the patient's functional oral-motor skills and their relationship to speech production and intelligibility.

Nutrition

A patient's nutrition is an essential area to be evaluated in home health, especially for the patient living alone. Awareness of nutrition problems or deficits is important, since poor intake can affect all aspects of the patient's rehabilitation program. The home health speech-language pathologist must be aware that changes in taste often occur due to stroke, and patients' reluctance to eat causes weakness and decreases endurance, strength, and production.

The clinician needs to know if a patient is on a special diet or is receiving nutritional intake from external sources, especially if the patient has swallowing difficulty. Table 4–3 shows some areas of nutrition that the clinician should examine. It must be pointed out that the speech-language pathologist does not examine these areas to provide treatment but to gain information and understanding in order to make an appropriate referral.

It is important to remember that nutrition plays a key role in the health of older persons and is important for their long- and short-term health. Good nutrition is important not only for maintenance of health but also for recovery from illness. Older persons should be referred to a dietitian if they (Squires, 1996):

- are diagnosed as needing a special therapeutic diet
- are not eating a full mixed diet
- are experiencing poor appetite or refusing foods
- are unable to maintain body weight/composition/biochemistry because of poor oral intake
- are overweight

Squires (1996) reports that a dietitian's nutritional assessment includes

- weight change
- hydration
- dietary intake
- clinical condition of the patient
- social assessment (e.g., home circumstances and mental condition)
- drug therapy
- biochemical profile/hematological measurements, if available or needed

Table 4–3 Nutrition

Evaluation Areas	Assessment Strategies
General nutrition	Appetite Hydration Diet compliance Enteral feedings Eating disorders Fluid restrictions New diet
Oral nutrition/diet	Regular Soft Pureed Mechanical soft Diabetic diet Calorie restriction Low-fat diet
Liquids	Thin Restrictions Thick Regular
Enteral nutrition	Nasogastric (NG) tube G-Tube Percutaneous endoscopic gastronomy (PEG) tube Other

Source: Copyright © 1997, Cecil G. Betros, Jr.

The dietitian's contribution to the management of home care patients with dysphagia can be a large asset to speech-language pathologists, who typically are not trained in the nutritional factors of the diets they recommend. The clinician should maintain a very close liaison with a dietitian, whether the dietitian is employed by the agency or on a consulting basis. The dietitian can be very helpful in developing interdisciplinary protocols for treatment of patients with dysphagia. In addition, a dietitian can advise team members on appropriate nutrition, following assessment of swallowing, and recommend types of foods for the diet. If the patient will be fed enterally, the dietitian can also advise on the appropriate feedings and the regimen, which are regularly reviewed and monitored.

Finally, dietitians can ensure that adequate nutrition is not only given to the patient but actually eaten by the patient. Speech-language pathologists who have worked in home health understand that diet compliance/noncompliance tends to become a major issue once the patient gets home. Families tend to want their loved ones to eat as they did prior to their recent illness. The nutritional value of food not eaten is zero, and therefore the food served needs to be acceptable, palatable, of correct consistency, and presentable to excite the patient's appetite.

Neurological Integrity

Speech-language pathologists working in home health must know basic history and assessment techniques to determine patients' neurological integrity. Regardless of the examination outline followed for the neurological assessment, there is no substitute for the knowledge gained by experience. The tendency is to see only those clinical findings that have personal clinical significance, and it is only with experience and development of a holistic approach to patient care that the list of significant findings expands.

An examination and observation outline that includes components borrowed from several different medical disciplines is presented in Exhibit 4–1. Specific neurological assessment techniques are not discussed here; however, the areas of observation are recommended, particularly for the beginning clinician, as a means of expanding awareness of each patient's neurological system and integration. Also, it is highly recommended that clinicians work closely with a neurologist before applying any techniques to patient care.

Exhibit 4–1 is not intended to be all-inclusive but is presented as a starting point for clinicians to use in observing the neurological conditions of patients in the

---

Exhibit 4–1 Speech-Language Pathology Inventory of Neurological Findings and Observations

• Numbness	• Confusion	• Unsteady gait
• Tingling	• Lethargy	• Vertigo
• Tremors	• Coma	• Neglect
• Paralysis	• Seizures	• Reflexes
• Sensory loss	• Vision problems	• Nystagmus
• Headaches	• Sleep disorders	• Side neglect
• Abnormal reflexes	• Weakness	• Pain

Source: Copyright © 1997, Cecil G. Betros, Jr.

home health environment. The component parts of the examination should be considered as questions that the clinician will ask regarding the patient's neurological status. If the clinician feels confident that he or she knows enough and has been properly trained, only then should any further testing be done by the speech-language pathologist. A word of warning: The clinician is not a neurologist, and information obtained from this segment of an evaluation is for information only and not to be used in diagnosis. But by conscientiously applying the observation and examination, whether by clinical observations or from the history, the clinician will learn to recognize subtleties of neurological pathology and will also have an organized approach to understanding communication disorders and related neurological dysfunction.

Speech-Language-Cognition

Protocols and diagnostic tests used in traditional settings are usually modified for patients in home health. Several factors influence the procedures of assessment in the home: the patient's endurance, the patient's attention span, background noise, and distractions. All of these influences can and do affect the type of responses and the validity of the test data obtained.

In addition, a process that should be looked at in any setting is that of function. The evaluation process in home health care is not just obtaining test scores and interpreting those scores; it is relating the scores to the patient's communication activities of daily living. Speech-language pathologists in general need to move from dependency on scores toward translating those scores into meaningful function or FCADL (functional communication activities of daily living). Functional outcomes are discussed in Chapter 10. However, functional communication is discussed subsequently in terms of evaluation and treatment planning.

A patient's functional ability is his or her ability to carry out daily tasks necessary to live. Many changes that accompany aging and disease make it difficult for people to be independent in performing daily tasks. A key word here is *independent*. In the past, speech-language pathologists have not looked at communication deficits in terms of dependence versus independence. However, in dealing with patients in the home, this becomes critical. No one—not the patient, the family members, or the health care professionals—cares if a patient can correctly point to a picture 75 percent of the time. What they do care about is how much better and more independent the patient has become as a result of that activity.

Speech-language pathologists must begin to think in terms of functional activities of daily living along a continuum from dependence to independence. Test scores must be translated into functional areas along this continuum. Thus, treatment must focus on the patient's independence in his or her environment, not on the patient's score on picture pointing. So, the clinician must think in terms of how

7/10 on an auditory comprehension test affects the patient's ability to live independently on a daily basis.

Table 4–4 gives some examples of how test scores can be translated into FCADL. Examining FCADL actually translates the patient's impairment into a disability. If the clinician can conceptualize that traditional test instruments used in the practice of speech-language pathology focus on the patient's impairment, not necessarily the disability, and grasp how the impairment disables the person to function in daily life activities, then function should become a natural assessment tool.

Table 4–4 Test Scores and Functional Communication

Test Area	Test Score	Influences on FCADL
Auditory comprehension	75 percent correct on pointing to pictures	What this says is that the patient is able to understand simple commands like "point to the block" with 75 percent accuracy. The patient will require some form of assistance with the other 25 percent in order to function. This assistance could be in the form of verbal cueing, repeating, or assistance with visual information along with verbal. Then the clinician can assess the patient's ability to understand conversation or follow simple commands (e.g., "Get your medicine").
Verbal expression	50 percent correct naming test items	Interpretation of this test score indicates that the patient is able to name test items with 50 percent accuracy. The patient will require moderate assistance 50 percent of the time. This assistance could be in the form of cueing, prompting, or initial sound recognition. The clinician then must assess the patient's ability to • call family members by name • name familiar household items • initiate conversation

Source: Copyright © 1997, Cecil G. Betros, Jr.

To take this concept one step further, disabilities result from impairments. To the practitioner working in home health, this means that the practitioner must be able not only to define the patient's impairment but also to define and assess how the impairment has disabled the patient's ability to live independently and carry out daily life activities.

The concept of independence can be used to assess the overall communicative status of a patient. There have been numerous scales and measures for independence, of which the most widely used and accepted in the medical community are those used by physical and occupational therapy. Although these scales are used to measure different aspects of disability, they can be easily adapted for use in communication disorders. Physical medicine and rehabilitation scales use the term *assistance* in relationship to the patient's ability to be independent. For the speech-language pathologist, the same principle can apply. Table 4–5 represents a rating scale for use by the practitioner in assessing a patient's disability.

Appendix 4–B presents an independent skills checklist that includes areas especially important in home health care. The list is by no means comprehensive but addresses some general areas of concern in regard to patients being treated at home.

Issues in Assessment

Methodological Concerns in Assessing Older Persons

The clinician faces certain methodological problems in assessing the older patient in the home. The clinician must be able to take a detailed history and obtain information relative to the patient's prior functional communication status in order to differentiate the effects of normal aging from those due to pathology. Therefore, the performance of an older patient needs to be compared with that of age-matched peers (Maxim & Bryan, 1995). The clinician must be knowledgeable about the effects of normal aging on communication and be able to ascertain the part those effects play in the patient's ability to communicate at the present level.

Very few tests of language and cognition functioning are specifically designed and validated for use with the older patient. Therefore, when using tests such as aphasia batteries, clinicians need to be aware of the test's validity, reliability, and norms. Timed tests especially will disadvantage the older patient. In differentiating other test variables, fatigue, poor attention, anxiety, background noise, and endurance clinicians must assess in terms of their effects on test responses and validity. Although these variables are present in a number of testing situations, they are very prevalent in the home situation. These variables can affect test performance and therefore must be appraised.

Table 4–5 Rating Scale of Disabilities

Rating	Definition	Modifiers
7	Preillness	The patient is able to perform the communication activity or behavior as well as he or she did before the current illness.
6	Independent	The patient is able to perform the communication activity completely but may be slow to respond; delays in processing could be exhibited.
5	Verbal cues only	The patient is able to perform the communication activity completely, but some verbal cueing may be needed intermittently.
4	Minimal assist/ cue	The patient performs the activity needing little assistance or cueing. At this level, 75 percent patient effort is seen.
3	Moderate assist/cue	The patient performs the activity needing occasional prompting or cueing; 50 to 75 percent patient effort.
2	Maximal assist/ cue	The patient performs the activity only with consistent assistance and/or prompting; 20 to 50 percent patient effort.
1	Nonfunctional	The patient is unable to perform the activity, even with maximum cueing and prompting.

Courtesy of Rehabilitation Institute of Chicago, Illinois.

Sensory deficits resulting from the normal aging process may also influence test results, especially those tests that rely on visual or auditory processing. For example, a patient's verbal difficulty in naming pictures may need to be distinguished from visual problems, that is, an inability to see the picture. Memory deficits can also skew test results in language tests that involve remembering auditory or written material.

Medications can also have an effect on the communication of the older patient. Older persons take many more medications than do younger people, and the effects of these medications are present longer as a result of a decrease in metabolic functioning. Although most speech-language pathologists rarely list a patient's medications, it is worthwhile to do so. The clinician should look up each medication and understand its effects, if any, on the patient's ability to communicate.

Drugs in the Older Patient—Special Considerations

Clinicians should have some knowledge of drugs and their use, abuse, and effects on communication skills. Speech-language pathologists should be aware of the most common drugs used by older persons and their purpose, and one excellent way to begin their education is to list all medications taken by a patient at admission. Other tips include keeping a *Physicians' Desk Reference* as a part of the clinical library and making notecards on medications, including adverse effects, purpose, and how the patient is to take them. The reference cards will come in handy and can be used as a therapy tool.

The following information is basic to pharmacology in relationship to older persons.

Compliance with Prescribed Drugs

- Compliance means taking drugs exactly as prescribed.
- For numerous reasons, 25 percent to 50 percent of patients do not comply strictly (Covington, 1995). Among these reasons are
  —cost
  —failure to understand the disease
  —failure to understand the importance of therapy
  —failure to understand the directions for use
  —number of drugs being taken
  —frequency of dosing
  —duration of therapy
  —relief of symptoms
- The consequences of noncompliance include
  —drug toxicity with overuse
  —therapeutic failure with underuse
- Approximately 3 percent to 6.3 percent of prescriptions are never filled (Covington, 1995).
- Medication should not be swapped with friends or family to treat symptoms that appear to be similar to those for which the drug was prescribed.
- Drugs should not be switched from the prescription vial to another container.
- Patients should consult with their physician or pharmacist before abruptly stopping any medication they have been taking for a long time.
- Patients should not prematurely discontinue antibiotics.

Adverse Drug Reactions

- An adverse drug reaction is defined as an effect of a drug that is unintended or undesired by the prescriber.

- Of all hospital admissions, 3 percent to 5 percent are due to adverse drug reactions (Covington, 1995).
- Prescription drugs most likely to cause adverse effects are
  –antibiotics
  –cardiovascular drugs (heart, blood pressure)
  –diuretics
  –central nervous system (CNS) drugs (tranquilizers, sleep aids, pain medicine)
  –hypoglycemics (Covington, 1995)

Some Facts about Drug Interactions

- A drug interaction is defined as the effect of one drug's altering the usual anticipated activity of another drug.
- One drug may increase or decrease the effect of another drug.
- Drugs may interfere with the absorption of another drug.
- Drugs may interfere with the distribution of another drug.
- Drugs may interfere with the metabolism of another drug.
- Drugs may interfere with the elimination of another drug.
- Drugs may interact adversely with certain foods.
- Drugs that interact can be given together, but patients should be carefully monitored for the need to make appropriate changes in the dose.

Five Questions To Ask about Medication

1. What is the name of the drug and what is it supposed to do?
2. When do you take it and for how long?
3. What foods, drinks, other medicines, or activities should be avoided while taking this drug?
4. Are there any side effects, and what do you do if they occur?
5. Is there any written information about the drug?

The assessment of older patients can be a difficult task, but assessments in different areas or modalities involving a very select range of responses should decrease errors of omission and eliminate these difficulties. Assessment, combined with a detailed history, a prior functional communication status profile, and skilled observation should enable the clinician to accurately describe the language pathology of the older patient. The following elements are important in assessment of older home care patients:

- detailed home assessment, including family/significant others
- detailed understanding of the normal aging process and communication
- detailed understanding and profile of the patient's prior functional communication

- detailed understanding and facts regarding the patient's premorbid lifestyle, abilities, and personality, and the patient's current functional status in these areas
- detailed understanding of the patient's current FCADL

After the clinician combines data from all the areas of knowledge to form a conclusion regarding a patient's language, the clinician will need to test and modify that conclusion to arrive at an accurate diagnosis of the type and severity of the language impairment.

The Diagnostic Role

At this junction it is important to note several things regarding the role of the speech-language pathologist as a diagnostician in home health. A large part of home health care nursing and rehab services is teaching. The speech-language pathologist can play a vital role in home education programs by diagnosing cognitive-linguistic deficits that would interfere with patient learning. Historically, the speech-language pathologist treated only patients with neurological diagnoses who exhibited an overt communication disorder. However, this author recently completed a study on orthopaedic patients admitted to a skilled nursing unit at a local hospital. The results revealed that 22 percent of the orthopaedic patients had significant cognitive-linguistic deficits that would warrant a referral for further testing.

Manual Muscle Testing of the Oral-Facial Muscles

The oral-peripheral examination presented in the following text differs slightly from the exams with which most speech-language pathologists are familiar. For years, clinicians have tried to quantify the oral-peripheral examination. At best, they have succeeded only in describing what was seen, but they have been unable to quantify actual muscle action or lack of action. Phrases such as "left facial paralysis" were about the extent of the examination results. With the onset of managed care, clinicians must be able to quantify a disorder and its effects on communication. And in the oral-peripheral examination, poor range of motion or muscle weakness is significant only if it impairs the patient's ability to communicate.

The techniques described in this section are borrowed from the field of physical therapy. Although manual muscle testing is an accepted form of testing in physical therapy and other rehabilitative fields, it is a rather new concept in speech-language pathology. Clinicians must learn to touch their patients and actually feel how the muscles move in order to make an appropriate assessment. In the home, the clinician has no sophisticated equipment and therefore must learn to use touch as a diagnostic tool.

A basic consideration in testing any muscle group is the validity of the testing and the reliability of the examiner. Careful observation, palpation, and stabilization are the essentials for validity in testing. *Palpation* is defined as the process of examining by application of the hands or fingers to the external surface of the body to detect evidence of disease or abnormalities in the various organs, and *stabilization* is defined as the act of making something, such as in this case a muscle or muscle group, stable (*Taber's Cyclopedic Medical Dictionary,* 1989). According to Daniels and Worthingham (1986), the patient should be asked to attempt to move the part of the muscle through the range of motion. The examiner should observe and note dissimilarities in the size and contour of the muscle or group of muscles being tested and the counterpart on the opposite side of the body.

In interpreting a test grade of a manual muscle test, clinicians must consider the normal variation in length, bulk, and shape of body parts in different persons. In addition, there are age and sex differences in strength, endurance, and psychological status of patients. Another factor to be considered in muscle testing is the cooperation and willingness of the patient to put forth maximal effort when asked.

According to Daniels and Worthingham*, the basic grades used in manual muscle testing are based on three factors:

1. the amount of resistance that can be given mainly manually to a contracted muscle or muscle group
2. the ability of the muscle or muscle group to move through a complete range of motion: a vertical movement
3. evidence of the presence or absence of a contraction in a muscle or muscle group

The examiner is to add a plus or minus to denote a greater or lesser amount of resistance than the usual terms applied to the grades. In the testing of the oral-facial muscles, positioning is not a factor, and only very fine movements are involved, with the exception of the muscles of mastication. Therefore, the explanation of grades that follows is general rather than specific in terms of any additional scoring, such as plus and minus. Grades that may be used, according to normal practice, are

Zero—no contraction can be elicited
Trace—minimal muscle contraction
Poor—performance of a gravity-decreased movement

---

*Adapted with permission from Daniels and Worthingham, *Muscle Testing: Techniques of Manual Examination,* 5th ed., pp. 2–4 and 151–164, © 1986, W.B. Saunders Company.

Fair—performance of the movement with difficulty
Normal—completion of the movement with ease and control

Normal and Good Grades. The amount of resistance required for a grade of normal or good varies with the individual patient and the muscle or muscle group examined. If the muscles on the contralateral side of the body are known to be uninvolved, valid information can be obtained by giving resistance to each counterpart before testing the involved muscles. Otherwise, the clinician must depend upon experience to make a judgment.

Fair Grade. The ability to raise a segment of a muscle through its range of motion against gravity appears to be a fairly specific accomplishment, and performance falls between the extremes of not being able to contract the muscle and holding the segment at the end of its range of motion against "normal" maximal resistance. According to Daniels and Worthingham, manual muscle testing in its simplest form centers on this concept, and the judgment and skill of the examiner are used to determine whether the muscle or group of muscles being tested is at a "fair" level of performance or is above or below it, and to what degree.

A fair grade might be said to represent a definite functional threshold for each individual movement tested, indicating that the muscle or muscles can achieve the minimal task of moving the part upward against gravity through its range of motion.

Poor Grade. The poor grade denotes the patient's ability to move a part through a range of motion on the horizontal plane, which can be termed a *gravity-decreased movement.* Although considered below the functional range, muscles graded poor provide a valuable measure of stability to a joint.

Trace and Zero Grades. A trace or an absence of a muscle contraction is determined by careful observation and palpation of the tendons and the muscle bulk. An increase in tension or a flicker of movement may be more easily seen or palpated in a tendon if it is near the surface of the body. These superficial muscles should be checked first, followed by inspection and palpation of the contracted tissue.

VITAL PARTS OF THE ASSESSMENT

Functional Status on Admission

The functional status of a patient on admission must be assessed to determine an adequate baseline for treatment and to assess the patient's functional outcome. In addition, the functional status on admission provides information in areas not necessarily addressed in a speech-language evaluation. The following are areas of functionality that should be examined:

- knowledge deficits about communication disorder
- safety of environment
- ability to complete self-care activities
- degree to which assistance/cueing is needed for communication
- risk for aspiration
- ability to complete therapy program (poor attention, can work for less than 25 to 30 minutes)
- ability to identify objects and people in environment
- coping/noncoping with disability
- nutritional deficit
- enteral feeding program

Significant Clinical Findings

The significant clinical findings portion of the evaluation is a brief summary of the patient's current presenting communication deficits. The report can be in the form of a short narrative or a list of statements. The clinician report does not need to be lengthy. A short summary of the clinical findings will suffice.

Skilled Treatment/Instructions on This Visit

Evaluation visits are not a covered Medicare service. The Medicare HIM-11 states that evaluation visits are a part of the admission process and therefore are not reimbursable under the Medicare program. As such, the clinician must be able to document that a skill was performed in addition to the evaluation in order for the evaluation visit to be covered. The following are some examples of skilled interventions that can be done on the initial evaluation visit:

- demonstration of neuromuscular exercises to patient or family
- teaching of safety techniques for swallowing
- presentation of a list of common words that the patient can repeat to make needs known

Patient and Family Goals/Perceptions/Expectations

More often than not, patient or family goals differ from those of the clinician. The patient and family usually have much higher goals. It is imperative that the clinician ask about the goals that the patient and family want to achieve. This provides a means of determining how well the patient/family understands the problem(s) and also sets the stage for counseling that the patient/family may need during the course of treatment. If the patient/family goals are unrealistic, the clinician must address this so that their expectations become more realistic. Often, patients and families become dissatisfied with treatment or the clinician because they feel that their goals are not being met, when, in actuality, the patient may not have the ability to improve at the level or pace they had anticipated.

The Need for Skilled Speech-Language Pathology Services

In this section, the clinician needs to document why the patient needs professional services. It is also important to define this need in terms of the patient's needing a skilled therapist and not skills that can be accomplished by the family or support personnel under the direct supervision of a skilled therapist.

CASE STUDIES

The following examples of actual cases seen in home health care illustrate the dynamics that can arise in home care and the treatment areas that can be addressed in the home care environment.

Case 1

An 85-year-old female was referred to the home health agency with an admitting diagnosis of cerebrovascular accident (CVA). In addition, the patient suffered a right hemiparesis and was "unable to speak or stand." The first purpose of the referral to the speech-language pathologist was to evaluate the patient's current communication abilities, that is, strengths and weaknesses. The physician initially requested an assessment with follow-up orders for treatment.

Assessment

Assessment for a patient with a left CVA and right hemiparesis involved receptive and expressive language, oral-motor movement, and swallowing. In addition, family and community resources were assessed.

Individual: The patient had received prior speech-language pathology services from an acute care hospital for two months and from a skilled nursing facility for two months. She was an independent communicator prior to her stroke. She had completed approximately two years of college.

Family: The patient lived with her sister and also had a sitter who assisted in the patient's care. They lived in an upper-middle-class neighborhood. The patient's sister stated that she wanted the patient "to talk more."

Diagnosis

Individual: The patient exhibited a severe expressive and receptive aphasia accompanied by oral and limb apraxia. Testing revealed a severe expressive aphasia characterized by severe deficits in volitional speech. She was unable to imitate single words. The patient's automatic speech was assessed with 60 percent accuracy. The patient was able to receptively identify pictures in a field of two with 50 percent accuracy. She was able to identify environmental objects to 50 percent accuracy. Her vocal quality was poor, and she was on a pureed diet with liquids.

Family: The patient's family and sitter demonstrated knowledge deficits relating to the patient's current communication disorder. The patient's sister was focused on having her "talk more."

Planning and Goals

Individual:

- Short-term goals
  1. To perform an ongoing evaluation to assess the patient's status and progress.
  2. To increase the patient's expressive language skills through patient counting and singing in unison with the clinician, imitating vowels, practicing family names, and reciting days of the week with 80 percent accuracy in nine weeks.
  3. To increase receptive language abilities through the patient's following basic 1 and 2 stages of auditory commands, identifying objects and pictures, and answering simple yes/no questions with 80 percent accuracy in nine weeks.
  4. To establish a home program prior to discharge, with patient/family education.
- Long-term goals
  1. To decrease expressive aphasia for social exchanges and communicating basic wants and needs through imitation and automatic speech tasks with 90 percent accuracy in two months.
  2. To decrease receptive aphasia for increased communication abilities with caregivers through auditory comprehension tasks and receptive identification of functional communication pictures and objects with 90 percent accuracy in two months.

Family:

- Short-term goals
  1. Support network members will demonstrate basic knowledge of aphasia and its cause and prevention.

2. Support network members will demonstrate the ability to interact with the patient in activities of daily living and in social interaction within her home environment.
- Long-term goals
  1. Support network will be able to observe the clinician on a regular basis to gain a general understanding of the therapeutic process to assist in carryover activities to facilitate functional communication.
  2. Support network will be able to demonstrate the home therapeutic program prior to discharge planning. This will be accomplished by having the clinician observe the interaction of the family/sitter in the application of therapeutic exercises and drills.

Intervention

Individual: During the course of treatment, the patient initially was showing significant improvement in her speech and language skills, both expressively and receptively. Throughout the initial periods of treatment, the patient exhibited altered states of alertness and responsiveness. She developed some gastric pain, and her physician prescribed Tylenol III to decrease the pain. This tended to sedate the patient and her responses decreased at times. Approximately one month into treatment, the patient began having bouts of gastric distress with diarrhea. This condition continued into the third month of treatment as she continued to have difficulty related to an intestinal virus and the prescribed medication. As her medical condition declined, the patient's responses to speech-language pathology also declined. She was unable to attend to task items. This condition became chronic. In addition, the patient developed contact dermatitis over her lower torso, which spread under her arms. The home health nurse was called to assess the patient's medical condition. The patient was then placed on medical hold because of her inability to respond to speech-language pathology treatment. She was eventually discharged by orders of the family and the physician.

Family: The patient was visited by the clinician as a follow-up approximately two weeks postdischarge. The clinician found the situation in the patient's home in disarray. The patient's physical status had declined, and the patient's family and physician had decided to provide the patient with no nutrition in an effort to stop the gastric distress and diarrhea. The clinician contacted the home health agency supervisor and reported the finding. The agency then referred the patient to hospice and social services.

Discussion

This patient and family situation was tragic in that the patient had obvious rehabilitation potential. She was obtaining some speech and language skills and, after one month of treatment, was progressing well with reports of intermittent emergence of spontaneous language. As the patient's medical condition declined, so did her ability to communicate effectively or even respond with an adequate level of alertness. It appeared that the family and caregiver were unable to successfully address the patient's intestinal distress. The family agreed with this assessment. The nursing supervisors were contacted, and the patient was referred to social services for hospice care.

Case 2

A 69-year-old white male was admitted to the home health agency with a diagnosis of CVA with a right hemiparesis and aphasia. In addition, the patient's nutritional intake was through a PEG tube because of obvious dysphagia. The physician's initial orders were for speech-language pathology to evaluate for treatment.

Assessment

Assessment for this patient consisted of a speech and language evaluation. In addition, a swallowing examination was administered to gain an understanding of the integrity of the swallowing mechanism and the patient's prognosis for becoming an independent feeder without the PEG tube.

Individual: Prior to the patient's current stroke, he was an independent functional communicator. The patient was independently employed prior to his CVA. He worked as a manager of a flower shop in a local community. Reportedly, the patient was hospitalized in an acute care hospital and then transferred to a rehabilitation hospital.

Family: The patient was currently living with his son and daughter-in-law following his stroke. At the time of the initial assessment, his family appeared very supportive and interested in pursuing treatment with him.

Diagnosis

Individual: Initially, the patient was found to be nearly an independent functional communicator. He showed moderate cognitive deficits characterized by difficulties with problem solving and orientation to day, time, and current events. He also exhibited some mild aphasia characterized by word recall difficulties and difficulty in answering WH questions. He showed some signs of dysarthric-type speech characterized by a reduced speed, strength, and range of motion of the oral-facial structures. He had a moderate to severe dysphagia and was currently taking nutritional intake through a PEG tube.

Family: The patient's support network demonstrated knowledge deficits related to the patient's current communication abilities and swallowing. The family's primary concern was that of being able to get the patient on a regular diet.

Planning and Goals

Individual:
- Short-term goals
  1. To use oral-motor exercises to increase the speech, strength, and range of motion of the oral-facial muscles for improved speech and swallowing.
  2. To increase orientation to time, place, people, and environment.
  3. To increase the patient's ability to answer WH questions and thus increase recall of personal information independently.
  4. To increase memory and auditory comprehension through following multistep directions independently.
  5. To educate the patient regarding safe swallowing procedures and precautions.
- Long-term goals
  1. To enable the patient to demonstrate mastery of personal information within nine weeks with 80 percent accuracy.
  2. To assess swallowing and provide appropriate intervention, as indicated on the basis of an upcoming medical examination of swallowing and a modified barium swallow.
  3. To enable the patient to process and understand complex instructions and questions with 90 percent accuracy within nine weeks.
  4. To improve overall speech intelligibility and oral-motor musculature mobility by increasing the speed, strength, and range of motion of the articulators.

Family:
- Short-term goals
  1. Support network members will demonstrate basic knowledge of the cause of the stroke and the patient's current level of communication.
  2. Support network will demonstrate education and knowledge of safe swallowing procedures and precautions.
- Long-term goals
  1. Support network will be able to observe the clinician on a regular basis to assist in daily therapeutic management and carryover activities.
  2. Support network will demonstrate knowledge of appropriate swallowing techniques and precautions as evidenced by observation by the clinician.

Intervention

Individual: This patient continued to make excellent progress during the course of treatment. Approximately three months into treatment, problems developed between the patient and the family. He became increasingly agitated and reported that the family just "laid around all day." He complained that they were not feeding him regularly. He wanted to leave and get a place of his own. During a follow-up modified barium swallow, the clinician conducted a family counseling session to see if the family problems could be resolved. A great deal of anger was unveiled during the session by both the patient and the family members. It appeared that the patient wanted to move into his own residence because the current residence was too small. The patient and family then moved and treatment continued. Eventually, the patient was able to remove his PEG tube. The patient was eventually discharged until his new location could be established.

Family: Although this patient's family remained supportive during treatment sessions, the patient was able to verbalize a declining situation when the clinician was not there. There was unresolved anger both from the patient and from the son and daughter-in-law. Eventually, a social worker was contacted and began to work with the patient in an attempt to aid the patient in finding an appropriate new residence.

Discussion

During this patient's treatment, he remained very motivated to improve his function of communication, graphic skills, and swallowing competency to live independently. The patient demonstrated very significant improvement in all areas of the treatment plan. The most significant improvement involved the eventual removal of his PEG tube. After a follow-up modified barium swallow, the patient was determined to be safe for liquids. He demonstrated excellent carryover of safety precautions and was able to take all intake by mouth. This patient was very motivated to improve his overall communication and swallowing abilities as he was quite focused on living independently.

The patient was eventually discharged because of the potential for a volatile situation to emerge as a result of the patient's desire to relocate. The patient decided to keep his desire to relocate confidential from his current "family/caregivers." During the course of treatment, the clinician had been questioned extensively by the patient's son regarding the need for a social worker and why the clinician was addressing the patient's writing and math skills.

This patient was eventually relocated to an apartment where he is living independently.

Case 3

A 76-year-old white male was referred to the home health agency with an admitting diagnosis of CVA with left hemiparesis. The purpose of the referral to the speech-language pathologist was to evaluate the patient's current cognitive-linguistic and swallowing abilities.

Assessment

Assessment for the patient with a right CVA and left hemiparesis involved receptive and expressive language, oral-motor movements, and swallowing. In addition, the patient was examined for visual-motor deficiencies and left field neglect. Patients with right-hemisphere damage are also examined for memory dysfunction.

Individual: The patient had received approximately one month of prior speech-language pathology services twice daily in an acute care hospital. In addition, he had received intensive physical therapy. He was an independent communicator prior to his stroke. During the patient's acute care hospital stay, he developed pneumonia secondary to dysphagia. He had a do-not-resuscitate order for approximately one week when he had a very poor prognosis. All therapies were discontinued until the patient's medical condition stabilized. Upon discharge from the hospital, the patient was placed on NG tube feedings. A modified barium swallow was not completed during his hospital stay because of the acuteness of his illness. When his medical condition was stabilized, he was discharged home.

Family: The patient lived with his wife of more than 40 years. They lived in a middle-class neighborhood. He had one son, who was not supportive of him or his wife but visited on an irregular basis.

Diagnosis

Individual: The patient exhibited a moderately severe cognitive-linguistic disorder accompanied by severe dysarthria of speech and oral-pharyngeal phase dysphagia. The patient was able to put together long connected segments of spontaneous speech. However, his speech often lacked psychological content. He had difficulty keeping on task and was not oriented. He had a severe left-sided facial weakness/paresis with a reduced speed, strength, and range of motion of the articulators. Moderately severe symptoms of oral-pharyngeal phase dysphagia were present, and nutritional intake was through an NG tube. No oral intake was provided initially. The patient showed severe left visual field neglect with poor orientation to visual-motor abilities, poor graphic skills, and a decrease in short-term memory skills.

Family: The patient's wife demonstrated knowledge deficits relating to the patient's current communication disorder. The wife was very anxious and at times showed signs of agitation. She was very concerned over the amount of hospital equipment being used, since the patient was initially bedbound.

Planning and Goals

Individual:
- Short-term goals

1. To use ongoing evaluation to assess the patient's status and progress.
2. To improve the patient's speed, strength, and range of motion of the articulators by administration of oral-motor exercises and massage techniques to the left side.
3. To establish cotreatment guidelines with physical therapy on improving the patient's motor responses and improving the patient's CNS responses to motor stimulation.
4. To establish cotreatment guidelines with occupational therapy regarding left visual field neglect and compensatory feeding techniques.
5. To increase the patient's oral intake of graduated (3 to 5 cc) thick liquids.
6. To increase the psychological content of the patient's verbal expressive skills by increasing his ability to respond appropriately and attend to task items.

- Long-term goals
  1. To increase verbal expressive skills for social exchanges and communicating basic wants and needs through automatic speech tasks with 90 percent accuracy.
  2. To increase the patient's speech intelligibility by decreasing dysarthria by improving oral-motor responses to oral-facial muscle exercises.
  3. To improve oral intake by introducing safe swallowing procedures and to remove NG tube feeding by addition of graduated oral intake of a variety of foods and food textures.
  4. To improve left-sided neglect by establishing cotreatment guidelines with physical and occupational therapy to establish awareness of the left side during treatment and in carryover procedures. Each therapy will be able to assist the other during treatment procedures.

Family:
- Short-term goals
  1. To establish a support network for the wife and patient. The support network will demonstrate basic knowledge of the patient's current cognitive-linguistic dysfunction and swallowing.
  2. Support network will demonstrate the ability to interact with the patient in activities of daily living and in social interaction within his home environment.
  3. Support network will be able to demonstrate safe oral-intake procedures by observing the speech-language pathologist.
- Long-term goals
  1. Support network will be able to observe the clinician on a regular basis to gain a general understanding of the therapeutic process to assist in carryover activities to facilitate functional communication.

2. Support network will be able to verbalize safe swallowing techniques and demonstrate appropriate feeding procedures and precautionary oral-intake measures.
3. Support network will be able to demonstrate the home therapeutic program prior to discharge planning. This will be accomplished by having the clinician observe the interaction of the family in application of therapeutic exercises and drills.

Intervention

Individual:

- *Speech-language pathology.* During the course of treatment, the patient made significant improvement in his cognitive-linguistic skills. In addition, the patient eventually was able to take pureed foods orally and the NG tube was removed by the registered nurse. The patient's response to oral-motor training showed a significant decrease in left-sided facial weakness and asymmetry of the oral-facial structures. This resulted in improved speech intelligibility and swallowing behavior. He also became better oriented to date, time, and place and was able to attend to therapy tasks for 30 minutes at a time. He showed some improvement in left-sided neglect as he was able to recognize his left side. Graphic skills to the right improved to the point that the patient was able to write his name and complete arithmetic activities.
- *Physical therapy.* Initially, physical therapy emphasized range of motion exercises to the left lower extremity to increase strength for sitting and standing. In addition, balance exercises to increase the response of the vestibular mechanism were added. The patient progressed in physical therapy to being able to transfer from bed to chair and maintain balance and strength in the lower extremity. Ambulatory activities were attempted; however, the patient was unsuccessful. Physical therapy was discharged with the patient still using a wheelchair.
- *Occupational therapy.* Occupational therapy activities centered around functional activities of daily living. In addition, the occupational therapist assisted the speech-language pathologist in teaching compensatory eating techniques. Left-sided neglect was addressed in addition to upper left extremity motor exercises. The patient eventually was able to complete dressing activities using his right side predominantly. He was able to complete all grooming activities except bathing independently. He was eventually splinted, as he got little motor return in the upper left extremity.
- *Nursing.* Nursing was responsible for the patient's overall medical condition, and the nurse served as team leader. Techniques for bowel and bladder training were completed, and the patient was completely continent of both bowel

and bladder. In addition, nursing monitored the patient's respiratory status for dysphagia treatment and removed the NG tube.

Family:
- *Speech-language pathology.* The patient's wife was able to observe the clinician on a regular basis. She was able to demonstrate the ability to communicate with the patient in activities of daily living. She was very diligent in assisting the patient in homework activities. She demonstrated the ability to feed the patient on a regular basis.
- *Physical therapy.* The patient's wife was able to complete range of motion activities to the left lower extremity. She demonstrated knowledge in her ability to transfer the patient from bed to wheelchair.
- *Occupational therapy.* The patient's wife was able to gain an understanding of the patient's left upper extremity weakness. She demonstrated abilities in assisting the patient in functional activities of daily living. She was able to change the patient's splint and assist the patient in upper extremity range of motion exercises.
- *Nursing.* The wife was able to verbally demonstrate knowledge regarding the patient's medical condition and medication administration. She was able to carry out home bladder and bowel training, and the patient was eventually taken off the Foley catheter.

Discussion

This case demonstrates excellent interdisciplinary care of a patient in the home. Cooperative efforts were shown among the disciplines treating this patient. The patient made excellent progress in all aspects of his treatment. Upon discharge, the patient was able to function in a wheelchair with only minimal assistance from his wife. It was interesting to note, during the course of treatment, that the wife became more agitated as she realized that her husband would not be ambulatory. She verbally expressed to the speech-language pathologist her anxiety over the situation. She would constantly state that "this is not the man I married." She was also very saddened that all the money they had saved for retirement travel was now being used to make their home wheelchair accessible. She stated on many occasions that she was not even able to go and visit her sister, who lived on a farm two hours away. The physical therapist was then called back in to train the wife in transferring the patient from the wheelchair to the car so that they could visit her sister and become more mobile. In addition, the home health agency was able to assist the wife in obtaining sitter services on an intermittent basis so that the wife could assume her weekly duties.

CONCLUSION

Providing evaluation and treatment services in the home has become a practical, cost-effective, and successful method to help maintain a patient's functional communicative independence. Evaluating and treating environmental safety needs; neuromuscular coordination; FCADL skills; and sensory, perceptual, and cognitive abilities are critical in the home environment. In addition, evaluating the need for other disciplines and services the patient and/or family may be in need of reflects the holistic approach to patient care and allows the speech-language pathologist to be a true clinician rather than a technician.

This chapter provides a general perspective, along with some specific ideas that work in the home health arena. Each speech-language pathologist needs to have his or her own specialized methods, supplies, and equipment to maximize the program. Family involvement, a patient's motivation, and community support systems, along with a creative treatment plan that incorporates those elements, will greatly improve and influence the rehabilitation success of patients with communication disorders in the home. Speech-language pathologists working in home health have a unique opportunity to help patients and their families to function well in their home environment.

REFERENCES

Covington, T.R. (1995). *Drugs in the elderly—Special considerations*. Birmingham, AL: School of Pharmacy, Samford University.

Daniels, L., & Worthingham, C. (1986). *Muscle testing: Techniques of manual examination* (5th ed.). Philadelphia: W.B. Saunders Company.

Maxim, J., & Bryan, K. (1995). *Language of the elderly: A clinical perspective*. San Diego, CA: Singular Publishing Group.

Squires, A.J. (Ed.). (1996). *Rehabilitation of older people: A handbook for the multidisciplinary team* (2nd ed.). London: Chapman & Hall.

Taber's cyclopedic medical dictionary. (1989). Philadelphia, F.A. Davis.

SUGGESTED READING

The American Occupational Therapy Association. (1995). *Guidelines for occupational therapy practice in home health*. Bethesda, MD: Author.

GAO study on Medicare's new prospective payment system flags potential hazards for older Americans. (1985). *Aging Reports*, 1.

Health Care Financing Administration. (1986). *Home health agency manual* (Publication 11). Washington, DC: U.S. Government Printing Office.

Pepper Commission. (1990). U.S. Bipartisan Commission on Comprehensive Health Care, final report (S. Prt. 101-114). Washington, DC: U.S. Government Printing Office.

Seibers, M.J., Gunter-Hunt, G., & Farrell-Holton, J. (1993). *Coping with the loss of independence.* San Diego, CA: Singular Publishing Group.

Summary of the Principles of Universal Precautions and Body Substance Isolation of OSHA's Bloodborne Pathogen Standards

PURPOSE

- To identify work-practice controls used to eliminate or minimize employee exposure to bloodborne pathogens and communicable diseases.
- To identify work-practice controls that promote safe and competent patient care in the home.

RELATED PROCEDURES

- Use principles of universal precautions and body substance isolation (BSI) when implementing any clinical procedures.
- STOP indicates that the home health provider is to review this procedure before proceeding any further with patient care.

GENERAL INFORMATION

Universal precautions recommended by the Centers for Disease Control and Prevention (CDC) and mandated in the Occupational Safety and Health Administration's (OSHA's) bloodborne pathogen standard focus on protection of the health care worker from bloodborne pathogens. These guidelines contend that

Source: Adapted from *Guidelines for Isolation Precautions at Hospitals, Infection Control Hospital Epidemiology,* Vol. 17, pp. 53–80, 1996, Hospital Infection Control Practices and Advisory Committee, Centers for Disease Control and Prevention.

all patients should be treated as though they have a communicable disease. This philosophy is congruent with the concept of BSI; it is an approach that is used by many infection control practitioners to reinforce and implement the concept that all body substances (i.e., oral and body secretions, breast milk, blood, feces, urine, salivary droplets or airborne spray from a cough, tissues, vomitus, wound drainage, or other drainage exudates), including nonintact mucous membranes, are to be treated as a potential source of infection, regardless of whether the patient has communicable disease. The term *body substance* rather than *body fluid* is used to emphasize that precautions should be taken with solids, such as tissue or feces, as well as with fluids.

EQUIPMENT

Personal protective equipment provided to the employee by the home health department includes the following:

- disposable nonsterile or sterile gloves and utility gloves
- disinfectants:
  1. chemical germicides that are approved for use as disinfectants and are tuberculocidal when used at recommended dilutions
  2. products registered by the Environmental Protection Agency (EPA) that are effective against human immunodeficiency virus (HIV), with an accepted HIV label
  3. a solution of 5.25 percent sodium hypochlorite (household bleach) diluted to 1:10 parts with water (Mix a fresh supply of bleach every day for effective disinfection.)
- masks, disposable cardiopulmonary resuscitation (CPR) masks, goggles, air-purifying masks, moisture-proof aprons or gowns, shoe covers, and caps
- leakproof and puncture-proof specimen containers
- sharps containers
- liquid soap, dry hand disinfectants (alcohol based)
- paper towels

OSHA TERMINOLOGY

1919–1930 Final Rule

Bloodborne pathogens. Pathogenic microorganisms that are present in human blood and can cause disease in humans. These pathogens include (but are not limited to) hepatitis B virus (HBV) and HIV.
Contaminated laundry. Laundry that has been soiled with blood or other potentially infectious materials or that may contain sharps.

Decontamination. The use of physical or chemical means to remove, inactivate, or destroy bloodborne pathogens on a surface or an item so that it is no longer capable of transmitting infectious particles; the surface or item then is rendered safe for handling, use, or disposal.

Engineering controls. Controls (e.g., sharps disposal containers, self-sheathing needles) that isolate or remove the bloodborne pathogens hazard from the workplace.

Exposure control plan. A written plan designed to eliminate or minimize employee exposure (required of all employers whose employees have occupational exposure that is identified in a job description).

Exposure incident. A specific contact with the eye, the mouth, other mucous membrane, or nonintact skin or a parenteral contact with blood or other potentially infectious materials that occurs during the performance of an employee's duties.

Occupational exposure. Reasonably anticipated skin, eye, mucous membrane, or parenteral contacts with blood or other potentially infectious materials that may occur during the performance of an employee's duties.

Personal protective equipment. Specialized clothing or equipment worn by an employee for protection against a hazard. General work clothes (e.g., uniforms, pants, shirts, or blouses) not intended to function as protection against a hazard are not personal protective equipment.

Universal precautions. An approach to infection control in which all human blood and certain human body fluids are treated as if they are infectious for HIV, HBV, and other bloodborne pathogens.

Work-practice controls. Controls that reduce the likelihood of exposure by altering the manner in which a task is performed (e.g., prohibiting the recapping of needles by using a two-handed technique).

PROCEDURES

Hand Washing

Hands are to be washed before and after patient contact. Wash hands during patient care if hands become soiled. Wash hands with soap and water immediately after removing gloves. Wearing gloves does not eliminate the necessity for hand washing. If soap and water are not available, antiseptic hand cleanser may be used. Then wash hands with soap and water as soon as possible.

Gloves

Don gloves before contact with nonintact skin or with blood or body substances. Wear nonsterile latex gloves when performing any clinical procedure that may expose the staff to the patient's blood or other body substances (e.g., during certain dressing changes or while inserting a urinary catheter). Utility gloves are used to clean up equipment, the work area, or spills.

After each use, sterile and nonsterile latex gloves are discarded in a leak-resistant waste receptacle, such as a plastic trash bag. Utility gloves may be disinfected and reused. Dispose of and replace utility gloves that are punctured or that show signs of cracking, peeling, or tearing, or other signs of deterioration.

Additional Personal Protective Equipment

This equipment is provided by the home health department for use in appropriate clinical circumstances, including the following.

Gowns, Shoe Covers, Caps. Wear moisture-proof, disposable gowns, aprons, shoe covers, or caps if clothing, shoes, or hair may be contaminated with blood or other body substances. Remove personal protective equipment after use, and dispose of it in a plastic trash bag provided by the home health department.

Masks. Disposable face masks are worn whenever aerosolization or splattering of blood or other body substances may occur. Dispose of masks after each use in a plastic trash bag.

When respiratory isolation is required, post a homemade STOP sign outside the patient's room. Instruct the household to wear masks when entering the room and caring for the patient. The STOP sign should alert visitors, including children, of the necessity to wear a mask when they are entering the patient's room.

Goggles. Goggles or safety glasses with side shields are worn when aerosolization or splattering of blood or other body substances may occur to the eyes. Clean the goggles with soap and water after each use. If the goggles become cracked or heavily contaminated, discard them in a plastic trash bag.

Disposable CPR Masks. Use disposable CPR masks if they are required to provide artificial mouth-to-mouth resuscitation or mouth-to-stoma ventilation.

Air-Purifying Respirator Device Masks. Consider using an air-purifying respirator device mask that is able to filter particles that are 1 micron in size, with a filter efficiency of greater than 95 percent of given flow rates of up to 20 liters per minute, when caring for patients with tuberculosis. These are obtained from the employee health/education department and must be specially fitted for proper use.

Sharp Objects and Needles

Place sharp objects and needles in a puncture-proof disposable container. A needle should not be bent, sheared, replaced in the sheath or guard, or removed from the syringe after use. Avoid recapping needles unless it is done through the use of a mechanical device or with a one-handed technique.

Sharps containers have the following properties:

- puncture-proof
- red in color
- labeled with a biohazard sign on the outside
- leakproof

Never fill sharps containers too full, enabling the contents to protrude out of the opening. Do not fill sharps containers over two-thirds full. In the home, store sharps containers on top of the refrigerator or store them in a place that is out of the reach of children. When they are nearly full, bring the containers into the home health department for commercial waste disposal, unless intravenous therapy services collect the containers for disposal. Sharps containers are to be clearly marked and dated "close date" using the biohazard labels. They are then transported in the trunk of a vehicle to environmental services for incineration.

Specimen Collection

Blood or other body substance specimens are to be placed in a leakproof bag and secured in a puncture-proof container during collection, handling, storage, and transport. Label specimens with the patient's name and identifying data. Handle all specimens carefully to minimize spillage. Place the puncture-proof container on the floor of the trunk in the vehicle during transport.

Personal

Eating, drinking, smoking, applying cosmetics or lip balm, and handling contact lenses are prohibited in patient care areas.

Miscellaneous

All clinical procedures are to be performed in a manner that will minimize splashing, spraying, splattering, or generating droplets of blood or body substance. Mouth pipetting or the suctioning of blood or other body substances is prohibited.

OSHA REGULATIONS

Infection control standards and policies published by OSHA will be accessible to all home health employees for reference. A copy of these regulations is kept in the bookcase in the home health director's office.

NURSING CONSIDERATIONS

Notify the physician of any signs or symptoms of infection in the patient or caregiver. See the list below. Instruct the patient/caregiver in applicable infection control precautions in the home.

DOCUMENTATION GUIDELINES

Document the following universal precautions on the visit report:

- implementation of universal precautions/BSI
- any patient/caregiver instructions regarding infection control and compliance with precautions
- other pertinent findings

Update the patient care plan.

POTENTIAL SIGNS AND SYMPTOMS OF INFECTION

- changes in the skin:
  - –redness or rash
  - –heat
  - –swelling
  - –weeping or drainage
- green or yellow exudates or drainage in the wound bed
- elevated temperature
- sore throat
- cough or change in sputum production or color
- fever, chills, or sweating
- nausea, vomiting, or diarrhea
- burning or painful urination
- clouds or filtrates in the Foley catheter bag
- tenderness or pain in a body part
- stiff neck or headache
- diminished breath sounds or wheezing on auscultation; labored respirations
- tachycardia or rapid pulse
- mental status changes

Independent Skills Checklist: Speech-Language Pathology

PERSONAL HEALTH

____ Knows medications by name and sight
____ Knows purpose of each medication and can verbalize
____ Takes medication on schedule and without reminders
____ Knows names and phone numbers of physicians
____ Makes physician's appointments without help
____ Knows emergency telephone numbers
____ Knows what information to provide when calling an emergency medical number
____ Can name and demonstrate use of first aid items and can locate them in house
____ Understands what should be kept in medicine cabinet, proper storage, and purpose of each item
____ Can name and demonstrate use of personal hygiene items

NUTRITIONAL HEALTH

____ Eats a variety of foods providing adequate nutrients
____ Avoids bingeing or purging
____ Eats at least two meals daily

Source: Reprinted from C. O'Hara and M. Harrell, *Rehabilitation with Brain Injury Services,* pp. 164–182, © 1991, Aspen Publishers, Inc.

SAFETY

____ Carries current ID

____ Can name and identify poisonous or dangerous products at home and their proper use and storage

____ Repairs items or can locate and secure appropriate repair services (phone book)

____ Knows location of smoke detectors and understands safety procedures during a fire

____ Can identify action to be taken after a robbery or break-in

____ Can locate and use telephone

____ Can name and demonstrate use of kitchen appliances

____ Can name and demonstrate use of hair care products

MONEY MANAGEMENT

____ Counts change accurately

____ Carries sufficient amount of cash or a checkbook

____ Understands how checking account works

____ Writes check properly

____ Keeps bank account balance in checkbook

____ Balances checkbook with bank statement

____ Understands how credit cards work

____ Knows total monthly income

____ Knows how to pay bills each month

____ Knows what financial assistance is available

MEAL PLANNING

____ Knows the difference between nutritional and junk food

____ Can identify various types of foods and which food groups they are in

____ Can develop a daily or weekly menu independently

____ Prepares shopping list

MEAL PREPARATION

____ Can name items of food to be prepared

____ Can prepare light meals safely

____ Uses sharp utensils safely

TRANSPORTATION AND MOBILITY

_____ Can ask for assistance when needed for walking
_____ Negotiates stairs safely
_____ Has current driver's license (if applicable)
_____ Can independently call for a taxi service
_____ Can give correct address and time for pickup to taxi
_____ Can independently make reservations for transportation
_____ Can indicate any special needs or physical assistance independently

TIME MANAGEMENT

_____ Identifies day, month, and time of day
_____ Arrives at appointments on time
_____ Keeps appointment book or calendar
_____ Independently records schedule in appointment book
_____ Independently checks schedule in appointment book

SOCIAL AND BEHAVIORAL SKILLS

_____ Responds appropriately to greetings
_____ Uses correct titles when addressing others
_____ Makes introductions appropriately
_____ Speaks louder or softer depending on situation
_____ Maintains eye contact
_____ Avoids interrupting others
_____ Responds to verbal/nonverbal cues and changes behavior accordingly
_____ Maintains conversational topic
_____ Expresses feelings
_____ Maintains comfortable distance from others when talking
_____ Responds appropriately to humor
_____ Exhibits facial expression appropriate to topic
_____ Demonstrates interest in others
_____ Demonstrates turn taking during conversations
_____ Shifts conversation topics easily
_____ Asks questions when needed
_____ Understands the concept of negotiation
_____ Demonstrates affection appropriately
_____ Follows rules at home

COMMUNITY INTERACTION

_____ Can locate numbers in white pages of phone book
_____ Can locate service numbers in Yellow Pages
_____ Can locate emergency numbers in the phone book
_____ Can make operator assistance calls
_____ Can take messages from incoming calls for others
_____ Posts or delivers messages consistently
_____ Understands the roles of health care professionals
_____ Plans and initiates activities

CHAPTER 5

Special Concerns in Home Care

The previous chapters have discussed and outlined some of the typical and modified speech-language pathology practices that are seen in home health care. This chapter discusses a few of the special settings, relationships, and techniques that the speech-language pathologist may encounter in developing a practice in home health care.

HOSPICE

Hospice is a specialized program of health care for patients who are terminally ill and their families. The goals of hospice care are directed toward palliation of pain and control of other symptoms rather than toward curative measures. Hospice care is appropriate only for those patients for whom cure is no longer possible.

The hospice program of care enables the patient to remain at home for as long as possible. Hospice caregivers encourage and support the patient and family to participate in decisions about the patient's care and to assist in caring for the patient. Each patient's family receives bereavement counseling and follow-up for a full year after the patient's death. This preventive maintenance allows the family to move on healthily after the patient's death.

An interdisciplinary team of specially trained caregivers, including physicians, nurses, pharmacists, social workers, clergy, dietitians, art therapists, physical therapists, occupational therapists, and speech-language pathologists, is available for each patient. An essential component of the hospice team is a group of specially trained lay and professional volunteers who support the paid staff and help to ensure the intensive level of high-quality hospice care. Each volunteer is integral to the success of bereavement follow-up for each family, and volunteers also support and augment the day-to-day care needed for the patient and family.

So, what is the role of the speech-language pathologist in working with patients who are terminally ill? Hospice care is certainly not the typical treatment setting and does not have the type of patients normally seen by the speech-language pathologist; however, the speech-language pathologist has a vital role in the care and assistance of those who are terminally ill. In accordance with the hospice philosophy of patient care, the speech-language pathologist helps to maintain the patient's communicative abilities and swallowing during the phases of the terminal illness.

Since adequate communication is required to carry out the goals and philosophies of the hospice concept of care, the speech-language pathologist becomes an integral part of the team (Betros & Downs, 1983). The speech-language pathologist must function in an expanded role to meet the needs of not only the patient and family, but other team members as well. The expanded responsibilities of the speech-language pathologist involve clinical intervention, consultation, facilitation of communication, and education (Exhibit 5–1).

Clinical intervention is a primary role of the speech-language pathologist in a hospice program. Because of their deteriorating physical condition, patients in the

---

Exhibit 5–1 Responsibilities of the Speech-Language Pathologist in Hospice

Clinical Intervention
- Address patient's need to communicate feelings of illness/death
- Improve patient communication
- Enhance communication among patient, family, and team

Consultation
- Advise team regarding communication of patient
- Advise family and volunteers of methods to enhance communication skills

Facilitation of Communication
- Assist in maintaining the flow of communication among patient, family, and team
- Participate in interlocking psychosocial process

Education
- Teach specific treatment methods
- Teach the professional role
- Teach methods to work with individual patients

Source: Copyright © 1978, Cecil G. Betros, Jr.

terminal stages of illness sometimes lose the ability to communicate effectively. Consistent with the philosophy of hospice, patients need to be able to communicate their feelings about illness and death with family members. One primary goal in clinical intervention with the hospice patient is improved patient communication, either verbally or through alternative augmentative communication methods. Although progress or improvement cannot always be achieved, communication among the patient, the family, and team members can certainly be enhanced. In addition to establishing forms of communication, the speech-language pathologist also plays a vital part in assessing the patient's swallowing abilities. Working closely with the dietitian, occupational therapist, and physical therapist, the speech-language pathologist can develop an intervention program designed to maintain the patient's oral feeding abilities as long as possible, which also helps to maintain the patient's dignity.

As a consultant, the speech-language pathologist is the specialist in speech, language, and hearing disorders and advises team members regarding communication of current patients. In addition to being a consultant to the team members, the speech-language pathologist also works with family members and volunteers regarding methods that can be employed to enhance communication and/or swallowing skills.

As a facilitator of communication, the speech-language pathologist's primary function is to assist in maintaining the flow of communication among the patient, family, and team. This is an interlocking psychosocial process that crosses all lines in a hospice program.

In the teaching role, the speech-language pathologist has many jobs, including teaching specific treatment methods, teaching the professional role, and teaching methods to work with individual patients. The role of teacher is most significant in that it can facilitate a better understanding of the speech-language pathologist's abilities and intervention strategies for the patient who is terminally ill.

Case Example

A 56-year-old white female was admitted to the hospice program with a diagnosis of progressive parkinsonism. At the time of her admission, the patient had a life expectancy of six to eight months. The patient was treated for three weeks before being referred to the speech-language pathologist. The referral to the speech-language pathologist was prompted by the family and patient, who were becoming extremely frustrated because the patient was unable to communicate basic wants and needs. The speech-language pathology assessment showed marked decreases in speech intelligibility and in swallowing safety. The speech-language pathologist started a program of therapy, to be delivered three times a week for three weeks, to increase the patient's neuromuscular control of the oral-facial muscles and to improve the patient's safety in swallowing. During the three-week period, the patient, family, and caregivers were educated in compensatory or augmentative communication systems for the patient to enhance verbal communication and allow the patient to make basic wants and needs known. In addition to alternative strategies for communication, compensatory strategies for swallowing were also initiated. At the time of discharge, the patient was able to slow down her speech enough to be understood. Likewise, neuromuscular integrity had improved with a home stimulation program. Both patient and family were also trained in a home exercise program. In addition, the patient was able to learn compensatory strategies for swallowing, which improved the overall proficiency and safety in swallowing. The patient was discharged approximately three weeks after admission to treatment.

Approximately two and a half months after the initial discharge, the patient was readmitted for speech-language pathology because of a decrease in communication skills. At that time, the patient's condition had deteriorated to the point where verbal communication was no longer an appropriate modality. A communication board was then established. The patient, family, and caregivers were all trained in the use and interpretation of the communication board. In addition, the patient had increased risk of aspiration due to reduced peristaltic action of the pharyngeal muscular tissue. Food consistency was changed to pureed, and the use of a percutaneous endoscopic gastrostomy (PEG) tube with supplemental oral feedings was recommended at that time. Again, services were provided to this patient three times a week for three weeks to establish the communication and swallowing system. The patient was discharged after three weeks with goals achieved.

Approximately four months after the second discharge, the patient was again admitted for speech-language pathology services. The patient's condition had deteriorated to the point of poor extremity motor control, which decreased the patient's ability to use the communication board. In addition, the patient was placed on a PEG tube as oral feeding was no longer an option. The speech-language pathologist's role at this time was to establish some form of communication system so that the patient and family would have some channel of communication available to them now that the patient was in the end stage of her illness. The speech-language pathologist saw this patient once a week to assess the efficacy and efficiency of communication and to make sure that there was an adequate communication system available to the patient. In the final days of this patient's life, the speech-language pathologist established a yes/no response system using one finger for "yes" and two fingers for "no." The patient soon died.

The hospice did an after-care survey, which asked typical questions, such as "How was the care?" "How did you feel about the care?" "Could things have been done better?" The most interesting finding was that the aspect of care that was most important to family members was that they were able to communicate with their loved one hours before she passed away. Of all the care the patient received over an eight-month period, the family most appreciated the care given to maintain the ability to communicate.

PATIENT AND FAMILY INTERACTION

In home health, speech-language pathologists have the opportunity to interact with patients' caregivers, families, and significant others. In other settings, the speech-language pathologist may see family members and/or significant others only occasionally, but in home health care, the speech-language pathologist sees family members on most visits; therefore, the speech-language pathologist must be able to identify family dynamics and the roles of different family members, and determine their effects on the patient's speech rehabilitation in the home.

In addition to providing the speech-language pathologist with a wealth of information, the family and/or significant others can play a major role in the total rehabilitation of the patient. Most family members are eager to learn ways to assist the patient in improving communication and/or swallowing; however, clinicians tend to be rather hesitant about using these individuals in the total plan of care for the patient. In general, most family members and/or significant others in the home are very adept at working on daily repetitive communication skills. Using their assistance frees the clinician from much of the "drill work," and being involved helps them to feel that they are playing a vital role in the patient's overall recovery. Teaching the patient, family, and/or significant other to do the repetitive day-to-day drill work for speech-language pathology will also allow the speech-language pathologist to address other issues that need to be dealt with during the treatment session, such as adjustment to disability, ongoing patient assessment, patient improvement, and so forth.

On the initial evaluation or assessment, it is critical that the speech-language pathologist determine the patient's and family's expectations and goals for the patient. If these goals are not addressed by the clinician, three or four weeks into the therapy, the patient and/or family may feel that the patient is not making enough progress, when, in actuality, the patient does not have the capacity to make as significant an amount of progress as they might have expected. Part of the clinician's treatment objectives must be to deal with family and patient expectations of therapy outcomes.

DISCHARGE PLANNING

For clinicians who work in an acute care setting, discharge planning can be a rather easy process in terms of appropriate placement and follow-up by long-term care and/or home care services. However, discharge planning for home care patients differs, since the patients usually will be maintained in the same environment. Discharge planning goals therefore tend to be different.

Discharge planning begins as soon as the patient is admitted to the home health care agency. During the patient's treatment in home health care, skills are taught to increase independence for discharge. The rehabilitation team helps plan for discharge. The word *rehabilitation* means to make able. The goal of rehabilitation is to make the person become as independent as possible. The rehab team consists of specialists in all areas of rehabilitation who will guide and teach the patient and family. The staff will help the patient increase independence (doing for self). In home health care, typically rehabilitation team members include the patient and family or significant other, a case manager (typically a nurse), a dietitian, an occupational therapist, a physical therapist, the patient's private physician, a social worker, and the speech-language pathologist.

Clinicians should maintain a list of national and local resources to assist with discharge planning. As the patient continues toward the goals of functional independence in the home and/or community, the following questions should be asked to determine training needs:

- What does the patient need to know to manage his or her illness or injury in the home?
- What will the patient be able to do? What will the patient not be able to do?
- What help will the patient need in activities of daily living?
- Will the patient need any special equipment? How does the patient get the equipment? How is the patient going to care for the equipment?
- If the patient is unable to be maintained at home, what are the patient's options at the time of rehab discharge?
- What are the patient's medications? Does the patient understand when to take them and know their purpose?
- When is the patient to see the physician, and at what frequency?
- Is the patient able to drive and do self-care activities?

Patient and family education by the rehabilitation disciplines also begins as soon as the patient is admitted. The team asks the family to learn and take part in all areas of care. This training helps the patient and family prepare for discharge.

The team conference in home health care usually differs from team conferences in the hospital setting. A team conference is a meeting of all the staff members of the team to discuss the patient's needs and to develop a plan. Since in home care the staff are out of the office visiting various patients, it is often difficult for team members to meet on a regular basis. Nevertheless, the most recent Joint Commission on Accreditation of Healthcare Organizations standards require a home health agency to have interdisciplinary team conferences for patient care. The first team conference is usually within the first one to three weeks of admission to the home health agency. During the first team conference, a probable discharge date is set, the frequency of visits of each discipline is determined, and terminal goals are established. This team continues to meet every 60 days, or as needed, to discuss the patient's progress until such time as the patient is discharged.

The most common conference type seen in home health is the family conference. Each clinical specialty is required to hold a family conference following the evaluation and then as needed. On occasion, however, a family conference—consisting of all the staff members, the patient, and the family—is required in order to discuss the patient's progress and/or lack of progress. During this meeting, goals are discussed and discharge planning, home visits, and family training dates are also reviewed and set. At this conference, the patient and the family can ask questions and talk about overall concerns of the patient. Not every patient will need a family conference.

Most agencies now require that some statement be made initially regarding the clinician's discharge plans. A discharge plan is more than a simple statement such as "discharge patient when goals are met" or "discharge patient to physician." Discharge planning means determining what the patient is going to be like at the end of the treatment when he or she no longer requires skilled speech-language pathology treatment. In addition, the clinician must determine what community resources will be needed, if any; what equipment or family education must be provided; and what home exercises the patient will need to learn to maintain his or her independence level as seen at the time of discharge.

THE PATIENT MANAGEMENT MODEL FOR DEVELOPMENT OF THE PATIENT PLAN OF CARE

Little or no literature exists that discusses the basic development of a speech-language pathology patient care plan or the process that clinicians need to adopt to effectively develop a plan of care. Most clinicians have used the IEP (individual educational program), which is basically an educational model, not a medical model. The clinician working in the home health care arena must develop the skills and understanding needed to develop a plan of care using the medical model.

Applicability of the Model

Of the many models, the most commonly used are those models that adopt a basic medical model of patient care planning; that is, they contain the following steps in some form: assessment, diagnosis, prognosis, orders, treatment, and evaluation of the treatment. While speech-language pathology can adopt the basic categories of the medical model, it has to develop its own terminology.

The medical model can be well suited to the needs of speech-language pathology in terms of patient care planning. Unlike the advanced nursing literature, which stresses the need for nurses to follow one or more parts of the model more stringently, thus indicating some problems with the use of the medical model, this is not typically so for the practicing speech-language pathologist (Stevens, 1983). In fact, there are very few, if any, problems relating the speech-language pathology care planning process to the medical model. For example, the categories of assessment and diagnosis are used in speech-language pathology in the same way that they are used in medicine. Like the physician, the speech-language pathologist assesses the patient through examination, which could be standardized diagnostic tests, physical examination, and history taking. Using the information attained in the assessment, the physician then makes a diagnosis, a process closely related to the speech-language pathology process.

Speech-language pathology uses the terms *assessment* and *diagnosis* in the same context as medicine does. More often than not, the speech-language pathologist combines all of the discrete symptoms into some further entity called diagnosis. If, for example, in patient assessment, the clinician judges that the patient has a deficit in visual perception, the clinician uses diagnostic assessment, goal setting, and care planning. Thus, speech-language pathology seems to differentiate, as does medicine, the two categories of assessment and diagnosis, whereas nursing assessment and diagnosis are not clearly distinguished. In nursing, the nurse uses the assessments as diagnoses in goal setting and care planning.

The medical model also associates prognosis and prescription and/or physician orders. The medical model dictates the following sequence of events:

1. Prognosis sets the realistic outcome to expect for this patient with this impairment.
2. To achieve the realistic outcome, or better, is the goal of therapy. The prognosis, in its form as the optimal realistic outcome to health, becomes the goal of therapy.
3. Prescriptions and/or physician's orders are then determined to reach the optimal goal. Such prescriptions or orders may be partial measures at any particular time, but they all aim toward the ultimate production of the goal.

In speech-language pathology, deficiencies in the areas of prognosis and goal setting are common. Outcome goals are seldom defined, or they are given in such broad terms as to be meaningless as a guide to physician's orders and/or final outcome criteria. The term *outcome goal* as used here means the final speech-language pathology goal for the patient, as defined in functional terms related to the patient's overall functional independence in the home. The outcome goal represents the ultimate realistic prognosis for the patient.

In many instances, and in most clinical practice settings, clinicians identify immediate goals before relating them to outcome goals and how these goals are going to improve the patient's functional communicative independence. The confusion appears to relate to the behavior modification model, in which a terminal goal would be that the person responds to a given treatment material 89 percent of the time over three sessions. The question is, how does such a goal relate to the person's outcome goals and make them more functionally independent in communication or swallowing? Clinicians, especially neophyte clinicians, have a very difficult time explaining what recalling three-step auditory commands has to do with the patient's overall increased comprehension and increased functional independence in the home setting. So, in essence, the care planning process needs to go one step further. The care planning process could include a statement that the patient should be able to carry out three-step auditory commands with 89 percent accuracy over three sessions, but the plan also needs to state exactly how such a goal affects the patient's overall functional abilities in the home.

Patient Assessment

Patient assessment in speech-language pathology combines assessment and diagnosis from the medical model. It usually involves, in one form or another, four techniques for assessment of the present and premorbid communicative status of the patient: a physical examination, standardized testing, clinical observation, and interview. The structure of assessment tools represents ways of categorizing the important aspects of human beings as well as speech-language pathology. Tools are used in assessment to make the process both systematic and complete. Clinicians vary in their philosophy and their process of assessment or diagnostic evaluations, but several commonsense rules can be applied to the evaluation or construction of assessment tools:

- The assessment tools should not duplicate investigations already available from other sources. There is no reason why clinicians cannot use for speech-language pathology purposes information gained by others. Unnecessary duplication of examinations or interviews is wasteful of the clinician's time and stressful to the patient.
- The assessment should seek only information that will be used in the care planning process. No matter how weighted the subject may be in relation to the patient's life, unless it will actually enter into the clinician's care planning, obtaining such information is an invasion of privacy.
- The evaluation form or reporting criteria should allow for discretion in collection of data. Compulsive form filling is not an appropriate use of the clinician's time. One of the most valuable parts of an assessment or a diagnostic evaluation may be the clinician's decision that certain sections of the

assessment tool are not pertinent for the patient and can be omitted without impairing the clinician's plan of care.
- The assessment tool should be realistic in terms of the speech-language pathology actually practiced or practicable in the literature.

Patient assessment, then, is usually a combination of assessment and diagnosis. Raw data are collected, but these data are selected through a preconceived screen of assessment tools that are based on the typical practice of speech-language pathologists in home care. To reduce assessment data to a workable size, clinicians normally use the method of exception in home health care. *Exception* means that only the communicative and/or swallowing problems seen as abnormal or deficient are considered in the diagnostic process. To identify speech-language and swallowing abnormalities requires that the patient's premorbid communication abilities and swallowing patterns be built into the assessment process. Both sets of criteria are very important in the clinician's overall ability to establish appropriate goals for the patient. The diagnostic and/or assessment data should be matched to the patient's premorbid abilities so that appropriate care planning may take place. The clinician must take the patient's state of adaptation to standing deficiencies into account in goal setting.

Goal Setting

Goal setting in speech-language pathology can be loosely equated with prognosis in the medical model. They are similar in that they both represent anticipated patient outcomes. The nature of these outcomes can be quite different, however. Medical prognosis is a practiced guess at the statistically likely outcome for the patient. Where the term *speech-language pathology prognosis* is used, it usually has a similar meaning (statistically likely outcome).

However, the clinician must understand that goal setting differs from the statistical observation approach to outcome. Long-term speech-language pathology goals define the desired patient outcome, given the realities of the patient's impairment. While prognosis aims at the statistical average, long-term goals aim at the highest level of outcome that can be realistically anticipated, given optimal communicative and/or swallowing return. This realistic goal setting requires both knowledge of the usual outcome for a given illness and the ability to estimate the patient's motivation, opportunities, and capacities. Thus, statistical and uniquely individual factors are combined in setting long-term speech-language pathology goals.

As in the medical model, a speech-language pathology prognosis is not further compartmentalized. The prognosis may change as the patient's conditions alter, but the medical prognosis is always a unitary concept. This too is seen in speech-language pathology.

Not only does goal setting involve multiplicity in content, but each goal is further broken down into goal stages. A good care plan will indicate short-term or immediate goals and show how each immediate goal is related to one or more of the long-term goals. For example, some immediate goals that might appear at one time or another on the way to the long-term goal of return to intelligible speech include the following: (1) The patient will have increased strength and range of motion of the oral-facial musculature; (2) the patient will be able to produce single words with 90 percent intelligibility; and (3) the patient will be able to put short, intelligible phrases together to make basic wants and needs known.

In evaluating the adequacy of goal-setting activities, the clinician should be aware of several sources for error in both long-term and short-term goal decisions: setting an inappropriate goal, omitting a needed goal, or setting an appropriate goal but for the wrong time.

Therapy Planning

Goal setting is translated into action by turning the immediate goals into orders for therapies most effective in reaching those goals. Speech-language pathology orders are the ongoing plans for speech-language pathology care: A speech-language pathology care plan represents the confirmation of such orders on a particular day. Orders for speech-language pathology need to be kept as permanent records in order to compare them with the permanent records of patient progress. Only in this way will speech-language pathology be able to research and evaluate its own process and its effects on outcomes.

Therapy planning is more complex than its medical counterpart, orders, because it must combine and coordinate speech-language pathology treatment and physician's orders. Although physicians rarely order specific speech-language pathology treatments or modalities, the reality remains that all care provided to a patient must be under a physician's order. So, a summation usually takes place in the form of a care plan. An effective care plan should be organized to show the relationship among the short-term goals, the long-term goals, and the expected outcome. In addition, the care plan must be highly correlated and show its relationship with physician's orders. Many traditional speech-language pathology activities are assumed to be the appropriate means for reaching certain goals on very little documented evidence.

Writing a comprehensive care plan for speech-language pathology is still a problem in many institutions, even though most speech-language pathologists agree that written care plans are necessary for quality care. The primary reason for care planning is that other health care professionals are now becoming much more educated in what the speech-language pathologist does. In addition, third-party payers also have become very knowledgeable in the treatments provided by the speech-language pathologist and the appropriate progression of patients to the end outcomes. The following are some additional reasons for patient care planning:

- Speech-language pathology as a profession must be willing to identify its own content, above and beyond the carrying out of medical orders.
- Agreement in approaches to speech-language pathology requires a written plan of care.
- Continuity of care from one clinician to another requires a written plan of care.
- Formulation of a written plan of care will help the speech-language pathologist to clarify and solidify goals.
- It is necessary to identify precisely the components of care in order to have a check against care omissions.
- Nonprofessional personnel need to have clearly established and well-communicated goals and outcomes.

Treatment Implementation

Treatment implementation is the phase in which the clinician provides needed treatment to meet the goals and functional outcomes. The treatment regimens for speech-language pathology have a complex structure because both speech-language pathology treatments and certain prescribed medical regimens must be implemented. There are two tools for the treatment implementation stage. One consists of the routing speech-language pathologist's charting, which is primarily a legal documentation system to validate the care given. It includes the recording of actual treatments given, the patient's response to treatment, home programming, any diagnostic evaluations, and so forth. These records primarily certify that selective care was given. The record of primary importance in the care or treatment implementation phase is the progress note. It is important that the progress note be just that—professional judgment of patient response to the related speech-language pathology therapy.

Care Plan Evaluation

Evaluation of the effectiveness of a care plan is an essential step in providing professional speech-language pathology in a medical setting. The two discrete parts of care plan evaluation concern the actual speech-language pathology treatments and the patient outcomes. The first part of the evaluation examines those aspects under the control of speech-language pathology theory and actual practice. The second part is the evaluation of those empiric changes that occur in the patient and are contiguous in time with the speech-language pathology treatments.

Evaluating the speech-language pathology treatment process involves a step-by-step analysis of the decisions made in each phase in the model. The model to be analyzed is the model used by the particular institution. For the model used in this chapter, criterion knowledge is identified in Exhibit 5–2. Every criterion knowledge would need to be developed into a set of standards in order to create evaluation tools for each phase of the treatment process. In this model, evaluation is needed of the accuracy of the patient assessment, the fitness of the goals selected, the adequacy of treatment planning, and the skill demonstrated in applying that treatment.

Analysis of patient outcomes is the second part of care evaluation. Patient outcomes need to be evaluated at various stages of the recovery process. Some illnesses or conditions present clearly defined stages; others require arbitrary definition of stages for evaluation purposes. As in evaluating the treatment process, evaluation of patient outcomes requires the setting of standards. In this case, criterion-based patient outcomes will need to be established to which empirical patient outcomes can be compared.

Relating patient outcomes to the treatment process is the final step in care plan evaluation. This is the area in need of much research and clearly is the area that offers promise for establishment of new and validated speech-language pathology treatment practices.

DYSPHAGIA MANAGEMENT IN HOME HEALTH CARE

One of the biggest challenges facing the home health speech-language pathologist is managing the patient with swallowing disorders. Unlike clinicians in acute care or outpatient settings, the speech-language pathologist working in the home does not have sophisticated equipment available for use in differential diagnosis. In many instances, patients confined to their home also have no means of getting to and from outpatient diagnostic centers for modified barium swallows.

Home care clinicians usually must rely on their own bedside diagnostic skills to make professional judgments regarding patients' swallowing abilities. Clinicians in home care also find it difficult to obtain diagnostic studies completed at other facilities. Therefore, clinicians working in the home must depend on their ability to diagnose swallowing problems and a patient's risk of aspiration without the advantage of the technology and equipment offered in other settings. Clinicians may find some useful guidelines in the overview of the dysphagia bedside/home

Exhibit 5–2 Speech-Language Pathology Plan of Care

Diagnosis: Moderate to Severe Receptive and Expressive Aphasia and Apraxia of Speech

Initial	Date	Problem	Short-Term Goals	Long-Term Goals	Outcome	Status
		Evaluation	Ongoing evaluation to assess communicative ability	Assess communication independence	Communication independence	
		Expressive aphasia	1. Produce single-syllable words in imitation, progressing to volitional production. 2. Produce bisyllabic words in imitation, progressing to minimal cueing from clinician. 3. Improve word retrieval accuracy in confrontation naming and sentence completion.	Improved verbal expressive abilities to the two-word level with 95 percent accuracy	Patient will be able to verbalize basic wants and medical needs to family/caregivers and other health care team members.	
		Receptive aphasia	1. Respond to simple yes/no commands by pointing to familiar objects. 2. Follow one-part auditory commands with 90 percent accuracy.	Increased auditory receptive abilities to the two- to three-part auditory command level with 90 percent accuracy	Improved patient ability to understand will allow patient to give more accurate verbal	

continues

Exhibit 5-2 continued

Initial	Date	Problem	Short-Term Goals	Long-Term Goals	Outcome	Status
			3. Follow two-part auditory commands with 90 percent accuracy.		information to family and other health care team members.	
		Apraxia	Strengthen volitional motor control of the oral-facial muscles to 95 percent accuracy for oral-nonverbal movements and syllable production.	Improved neuromuscular control and strength of the oral-facial muscles	Improved speech intelligibility and understanding by family and others	
		Safety	Patient will be able to make medical needs known by one-word utterance supplemented by augmentative communication.	1. Understand and identify all medications. 2. Understand all teaching materials given by other team members. 3. Be able to verbalize and/or gesture understanding of the home education program (HEP).	Improved safety within the home environment	

continues

Exhibit 5–2 continued

Initial	Date	Problem	Short-Term Goals	Long-Term Goals	Outcome	Status
		Home exercise program	1. Neuromuscular exercises 2. Identification of familiar objects	Use augmentative communication system to supplement verbal and auditory communication skills.	Established HEP for maintenance of current skills	
		Patient/family education	1. Causes of stroke 2. Stroke prevention 3. Communication difficulties associated with stroke 4. Conference regarding evaluation results and prognosis	1. Health maintenance and prevention of stroke 2. Reinforcement of education from other disciplines	Patient and family will be educated on stroke and stroke prevention.	
		Patient and family goals	1. Determine therapeutic expectations following assessment. 2. Establish written patient/family goals.	1. Decrease anxiety regarding communication abilities. 2. Provide counseling regarding patient progress and expected outcomes and prognosis.	Patient and family will be counseled regarding therapeutic goals and their expected outcomes in order to facilitate a better understanding and acceptance of residual deficits.	

continues

Exhibit 5–2 continued

Initial	Date	Problem	Short-Term Goals	Long-Term Goals	Outcome	Status
		Discharge planning	1. Following evaluation, discharge expectations will be established with patient and family. 2. Evaluate patient status every 60 days to determine progress toward terminal goals and acceptance of residual problems.	Patient will be discharged as outcomes are reached. Patient will be a limited communicator who will need cueing for verbal output.	At the end of this treatment, the patient will be able to make wants and medical needs known to family and others.	

Courtesy of Communication Concepts and Consulting, Inc., Birmingham, Alabama.

health examination (Appendix 5–A). The examination criteria and outline are not meant to be all-inclusive. Although there has been no documentation in the literature regarding these procedures, they have been taken, partly, from experts in the field of swallowing disorders.

CONCLUSION

This chapter has attempted to show some of the special issues clinicians may encounter as they practice in home health care. Speech-language pathologists should be aware of the variety of treatment needs and settings of patients in the home environment and the special relationships that can develop. Dysphagia management is a special concern, since clinicians must be able to diagnose swallowing problems without instrumentation in most cases.

REFERENCES

Betros, C.G., & Downs, M.J. (1983). The interdisciplinary health care team. *Journal of the Speech and Hearing Association of Alabama* (Spring).

Stevens, B.J. (1983). *First-line patient care management* (2nd ed.). Rockville, MD: Aspen Publishers.

SUGGESTED READING

Huckabay, L.B.D., & Neal, M.C. (1979). The nursing care plan problem. *Journal of Nursing Administration, 9* (12), 36.

King, I.M. (1981). *A theory for nursing: Systems, concepts, process.* New York: John Wiley & Sons.

Krieger, D. (1981). *Foundations for holistic health nursing practices: The renaissance nurse.* Philadelphia: J.B. Lippincott Co.

LaMonica, E.L. (1979). *The nursing process: A humanistic approach.* Menlo Park, CA: Addison-Wesley Publishing Co.

Lash, A.A. (1981). Nursing diagnosis: Some comments on the gap between theory and practice. In J.C. McCloskey & H.K. Grace (Eds.), *Current issues in nursing.* Boston: Blackwell Scientific Publications.

Logemann, J.A. (1993). *Evaluation and treatment of swallowing disorders.* San Diego, CA: College Hill Press.

Logemann, J.A. (1993). *Manual for videofluorographic study of swallowing.* Austin, TX: PRO-ED.

Mackay, C., & Ault, L.D. (1977). A systematic approach individualizing nursing care plans. *Journal of Nursing Administration, 7,* (1), 39.

Orem, D.E. (1971). *Nursing: Concepts of practice.* New York: McGraw-Hill.

Parse, R.R. (1981). *Man–living health: A theory of nursing.* New York: John Wiley & Sons.

Phillips, J.R. (1977). Nursing systems and nursing models. *Image, 9,* (1), 4.

Reihl, J.P., & Roy, C. (1980). *Conceptual models for nursing practice* (2nd ed.). New York: Appleton-Century-Crofts.

Stevens, B.J. (1979). *Nursing theory: Analysis, application, evaluation.* Boston: Little, Brown and Company.

Woody, M., & Mallison, M. (1973). The problem-oriented system for patient-centered care. *American Journal of Nursing, 73* (7), 1168.

Home Health Examinations and Treatment

DYSPHAGIA BEDSIDE EXAMINATION

PURPOSE

To provide a formal and systematic method for performing a dysphagia examination in the home.

OBJECTIVE

To assist the clinician in evaluating patients who exhibit a swallowing disorder.

INFECTION CONTROL

The dysphagia bedside/home health examination is considered a category I activity.

POLICY

- Specialized training is needed by the speech-language pathologist to effectively administer this procedure.
- Only a licensed speech-language pathologist is qualified to evaluate the patient for this treatment procedure.
- Only a licensed speech-language pathologist is qualified to perform these techniques and document the results once the parameters have been determined.

Source: Data from J. Logemann, *Evaluation and Treatment of Swallowing Disorders,* © 1993, College Hill Press; and J. Logemann, *Manual for Videofluorographic Study of Swallowing,* © 1993, PRO–ED.

EQUIPMENT

- Sterile gloves (as needed)
- Stethoscope
- Penlight
- Tongue depressor
- 00 laryngeal mirror (sterile)
- 4 × 4 gauze
- Straws
- Syringe
- Food consistencies/textures
- Spoon

PROCEDURE

PROCEDURAL CONSIDERATIONS

1. Wash hands and put on gloves as needed.
2. Instruct patient/family on procedure to be performed.
3. **Take patient history:**
   Duration of swallowing problem
   Initial symptoms
   Better now?
   Food sticking in mouth?   Delayed reflex or reduced peristalsis
   Food catching high in throat?   Cricopharyngeal dysfunction
   Food catching low in throat?
   Coughing:
      (Can't tell when)   Reduced lingual control or delayed reflex
      Before swallow   Reduced laryngeal closure
      During swallow   Reduced peristalsis or cricopharyngeal dysfunction

   After swallow
   Current symptoms
   Current nutritional intake:
      Oral
      Nasogastric tube
      Pharyngostomy
      Esophagostomy
      Gastrostomy
      Jejunostomy
      Date nonoral feeding began

Current respiratory status:
  Tracheostomy tube: cuffed,
    uncuffed
  Fenestrated, unfenestrated
  Cuff deflated at times
  Date tracheostomy tube
    placed
Does problem vary with
  food consistencies?
Easiest consistencies

Suction mouth; remove inner cannula and clean. Complete deep suction as needed. Deflate cuff; suction trans-tracheostomy. Occlude tracheostomy during swallows. Suction after swallowing; reinflate cuff.

Use these consistencies later in trial swallows.

4. **Perform physical examination:**
During the physical examination, the clinician should evaluate not only the structure and function of the oral-facial swallowing mechanisms, but also strength and endurance of the musculature.

Oral Examination—Structure
The oral structures are examined for any abnormalities, and the clinician is to give a detailed explanation. Examine lips, teeth (maxillary), teeth (mandibular), tongue, floor of mouth, cheeks, faucial arches, tonsils, hard palate, uvula, and posterior pharyngeal wall.

Oral Awareness and Reaction
Introduce gauze, burlap, satin soaked with liquids of various flavors, temperatures; stroke lips, tongue (center and sides), buccal areas.

Identify stimuli causing movements used in swallow. Identify stimuli/areas of contact resulting in abnormal oral reflexes.

Chewing
Introduce gauze roll and assess lateralization and chewing.

**Oral Examination—
Function**
Labial
Range of motion
Lip spread /i/
Lip rounding /u/
Asymmetry: right/left
Lip closure at rest
Lip closure on repeated /pa/
Lip closure during sentence
repetition: "Please put the
papers on the back door."

Physiologically, patients often have reduced lip closure during chewing and
swallowing. To compensate for this, tilt
the patient's head slightly backward and
toward the stronger side to keep food in
the mouth.

Lingual
Range of motion
Elevation of tip
Elevation of back
Point to right side
Point to left side
Retraction
Asymmetry: right/left
Rapid repetitive lateraliza-
tion
Rapid repetitive elevation
Tip-alveolar contact on
repeated /ta/
Tip-alveolar contact during
sentence repetition: "Take
time to talk to them."
Fine lingual shaping during
sentence repetition: "Say
something nice to Susan
on Sunday."
Back-velar contact on
repetitive /k/
Back-velar contact during
sentence repetition: "Can
you go get the garbage
cans?"

Velar Function
Elevation on prolonged /a/
Retraction on prolonged /a/
Symmetrical movement

Oral Sensitivity
Light touch—tongue tip   Have patient close eyes and use a cotton-
Light touch—left side   tip applicator to stimulate.
  Lateral margin of tongue
  Posterior tongue
  Anterior faucial arch
  Cheek
Light touch—right side
  Lateral margin of tongue
  Posterior tongue
  Anterior faucial arch
  Cheek

Oral Reflexes
Gag   Stimulate base of tongue and posterior
                                      pharyngeal wall. Caution for patients
                                      who have hypersensitive gag reflexes:
                                      They will vomit.
Palatal reflexes   Stimulate anterior portion of soft palate.

Laryngeal Examination
Voice quality
Strength of voluntary cough
Strength of throat clearing
Clarity of /h/ and /a/ during
  repetitive /ha/
Pitch range
Loudness range
Phonation time

Pharyngeal Swallow
Delayed
Not delayed

Cervical Auscultation
See cervical auscultation
techniques.

Palpation
See palpation techniques.

5. **Trial swallows:**
From the history, the clinician should determine which consistencies are the easiest for the patient to swallow.

Begin with 1/3 teaspoon or 5 cc in a syringe. Patient can be progressed in food textures and amounts unless aspiration is detected. At that time, test should be terminated.

The following observations and notes should be made during trial swallows:
Lip closure during chewing/swallow
Tongue/palate contact
Tongue lateralization for chewing
Tongue/palate contact during oral transit
Lingual propulsion pattern
Control of bolus
Reduced tongue movement
Reduced oral propulsion
Velar closure during swallow
Loss of food in oral cavity
Pharyngeal peristalsis
Aspiration during swallowing
Reduced laryngeal elevation
Delay in pharyngeal swallow

6. Following the completion of the examination, a complete description of the results must be given to the patient/caregiver.
7. Explicit written instructions are to be left in the home for swallowing precautions and safe swallowing techniques.
8. The clinician must have patient and/or caregiver demonstrate the appropriate techniques left in the home.
9. Remove and dispose of gloves and protective eyewear.
10. Wash hands.
11. Document.

Include:
Procedure performed
Patient's response to procedure performed
Instructions given to patient or caregiver
Signature, date, time

Standard Treatment Time: 30–45 minutes, depending on patient's severity and speed of responses

CERVICAL AUSCULTATION

PURPOSE

To provide a formal and systematic method for performing cervical auscultation for the diagnosis of dysphagia.

OBJECTIVE

To assist the clinical practitioner in the differential diagnosis of dysphagia in the absence of appropriate radiological equipment.

INFECTION CONTROL

Cervical auscultation is considered a category III activity.

POLICY

- Specialized training is needed to effectively determine if a patient has a swallowing disorder and to appropriately assess the possibility that a patient is aspirating.
- Only a licensed speech-language pathologist is qualified to evaluate the patient, using cervical auscultation, for possible dysphagia.
- Only a licensed speech-language pathologist may perform these techniques and document the results once the parameters have been determined.

EQUIPMENT

- Stethoscope
- Nonsterile gloves (as needed)

PROCEDURE

1. Wash hands and put on gloves as needed.
2. Instruct patient/family on technique to be performed.
3. Auscultate both sides (independently) of the neck at the level of the larynx or directly under the mandible.
4. Have the patient swallow consistencies of thin liquids, thick liquids, or small amounts of solid foods.
5. Listen for signs of gurgling, wheezing, or rails.

6. Note any abnormal sounds and the side they were on (or bilaterally).
7. Remove and dispose of gloves (if used).
8. Wash hands.
9. Document. Include:
   Procedure performed
   Patient's response to procedure performed
   Instructions to patient/family
   Signature, date, and time

Standard Treatment Time: 20–30 minutes

PALPATION OF THE SWALLOWING MECHANISM

PURPOSE

To provide a formal and systematic method for performing palpation techniques to assist the speech-language pathologist in the differential diagnosis of dysphagia at bedside.

OBJECTIVE

To assist the clinical practitioner in assessing the movement of the laryngeal mechanism, strap muscles of the masticatory mechanism, and tongue during the act of swallowing.

INFECTION CONTROL

Palpation is considered a category III activity.

POLICY

- Specialized training is needed to effectively determine if a patient has a swallowing disorder and to appropriately assess the possibility of dysphagia.
- Only a licensed speech-language pathologist is qualified to evaluate the patient, using palpation, for possible dysphagia.
- Only a licensed speech-language pathologist may perform these techniques and document the results once the parameters have been determined.

EQUIPMENT

- Nonsterile gloves (as needed)

PROCEDURE

1. Wash hands and put on gloves as needed.
2. Instruct patient and family on technique to be performed.
3. With both hands, palpate the neck muscles when the patient is asked to swallow.
4. The clinician should note the movement or lack of movement of the laryngeal mechanism to the upward and anterior position.

5. The clinician should note the speed of the laryngeal mechanism as the swallowing act is being performed. Any time > 1 second should be noted and reported as a delay in the swallowing mechanism, which would put a patient at risk for aspiration.
6. Particular attention should be paid to the area of the posterior portions of the mandible during swallowing. Abnormal movement or a delay in movement could be indicative of poor posterior lingual control or movement, which could indicate poor bolus propulsion into the esophagus.
7. Remove and dispose of gloves (as needed).
8. Wash hands.
9. Document. Include:
   Procedure performed
   Patient's response to procedure performed
   Instructions to patient and family
   Signature, date, and time

Standard Treatment Time: 15 minutes

TREATMENT OF DYSPHAGIA WITH ASPIRATION

PURPOSE

To provide a formal and systematic method for managing patients with dysphagia and aspiration in the home.

OBJECTIVE

To increase the ability of the patient with aspiration problems to be treated safely in the home.

INFECTION CONTROL

Dysphagia management with aspiration is considered a category II activity.

POLICY

- Specialized training is needed to effectively determine the needs of the patient with aspiration problems.
- Only a licensed speech-language pathologist is qualified to manage the patient with aspiration difficulties.
- These techniques can be performed only by or under the direct supervision of a licensed speech-language pathologist.

EQUIPMENT

- Stethoscope
- Nonsterile gloves (if needed)

PROCEDURE

1. Wash hands and put on gloves (if needed).
2. Assess the patient's diet and make diet changes for safe oral intake.
3. Consult with patient's physician on alternative feeding programs.

SPECIAL CONSIDERATIONS

Often patients seen in the home have not had a modified barium swallow. The clinician should be proficient in bedside evaluation of dysphagia.

If a patient is aphasic, always insist on a PEG tube for alternative feeding program.

4. Swallow precautions:
   Bed positioning
   Check temperature every two
      weeks
   Cervical auscultation
   Nurse to check chest sounds
5. Indirect treatment would consist of oral-motor exercises,
   thermal stimulation with minimum oral intake, progressing
   as patient can tolerate.
6. Remove and dispose of gloves
   (if used).
7. Wash hands.
8. Document. Include:
   Procedure performed
   Patient's response to procedure performed
   Instructions to patient/family
   Signature, date, and time

Standard Treatment Time: 20–30 minutes, unless the patient's signs and symptoms indicate alteration of the treatment time

TREATMENT OF DYSPHAGIA WITH NO ASPIRATION

PURPOSE

To provide a formal and systematic method for the patient/family to acquire skills in safely managing the patient with dysphagia in the home.

OBJECTIVE

To increase the patient/family's ability to safely manage the patient with dysphagia in the home.

INFECTION CONTROL

Dysphagia management without aspiration is considered a category I activity.

POLICY

- Specialized training is needed to effectively determine the needs of the patient/family and their ability to manage the patient with dysphagia in the home.
- Only a licensed speech-language pathologist is qualified to evaluate the management of the patient with dysphagia and determine the parameters of management.
- These procedures may be performed only by or under the direct supervision of a licensed speech-language pathologist.

EQUIPMENT

- Sterile gloves (if needed)
- Tongue depressor
- Lemon glycerin swabs
- Oral thermometer
- Stethoscope

PROCEDURE

1. Wash hands and put on gloves (if needed).
2. Implement oral-motor techniques.
3. Implement thermal stimulation techniques.

SPECIAL CONSIDERATIONS

4. To increase posterior tongue movements, have patient produce /k/ and /g/ sounds or words.
5. Modify diet as needed or tolerated.

For patients that are at high risk for aspiration

6. Modify liquids/textures as needed or tolerated.
7. Implement protocol for positioning and swallowing precautions.
8. To increase sensation if the patient exhibits a facial droop, stroke affected side with ice or cold rag with ice.
9. Repeat as needed.
10. Remove and dispose of gloves (if used).
11. Wash hands.
12. Document. Include:
    Procedure performed
    Patient's response to procedure performed
    Instructions given to patient/family
    Signature, date, and time

Aspiration precautions:
Choking
Wet voice quality
Patient complaints of food or liquids being caught in throat

Standard Treatment Time: 20–30 minutes, unless the patient's signs and symptoms indicate alteration of the treatment time

PART III

Documentation, Reimbursement, and Accountability

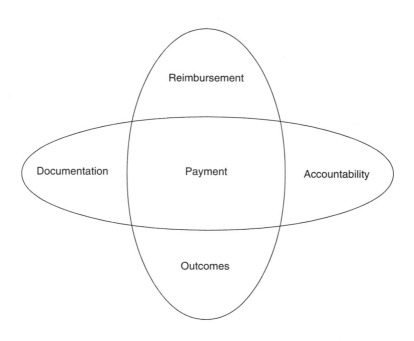

CHAPTER 6

Business Aspects of Home Care for the Speech-Language Pathologist

EMPLOYEE VERSUS INDEPENDENT CONTRACTOR STATUS

Over the past decade, the rapid growth of the home health industry has created a need for a variety of services for home care patients. Speech-language pathology plays an important role in total rehabilitation, since it allows individuals receiving services to obtain their maximum level of independence in the home. As more speech-language pathology practitioners enter the home care treatment setting to practice, the profession and the home health industry must develop a working relationship to meet each other's needs and still satisfy their own. The speech-language pathologist and the home health care agency both have responsibilities when entering into this relationship, and various types of agreements may be negotiated at the beginning of these work relationships.

Home health agencies can provide speech-language pathology services to their patients by hiring speech-language pathologists as full-time or part-time employees, or they may hire them as independent contractors. The latter method has become more common in recent years.

In some situations, speech-language pathology practitioners who practice as independent contractors may be in conflict with Medicare regulations. It is suggested that speech-language pathology practitioners discuss their specific job responsibilities with the home health agency and clarify the different parameters for speech-language pathologists practicing as independent contractors or identified as employees. It is important that each party have an appreciation and understanding of the other's limits, given the parameters of third-party reimbursement for agency costs and regulations defining independent contractor relationships.

The use of speech-language pathologists as independent contractors has advantages for both the home health agency and the practitioner. For the home health agency, it is cost effective because there is no need to provide benefits, leave, or equipment or to withhold taxes. Further, the home health agency can expand or reduce staff to meet its needs without making an expensive commitment to full-time employees. Independent contractors maintain high levels of productivity, and the home health agency is reimbursed for their services by third-party payers at a rate that includes the practitioners' fees and the agency's overhead, up to a limit. Thus, the cost of providing speech-language pathology services is usually completely funded by third-party reimbursement.

For practitioners, working as an independent contractor can offer tremendous flexibility and independence, which are particularly important to individuals interested in raising a family while maintaining a job and to those who desire more free time. Independent contractors should be responsible for their own scheduling—choosing their own hours and determining when they will treat their clients. In addition, speech-language pathologists can benefit from many other advantages of having their own private practice. These benefits may include such amenities as tax write-offs (a review of the most recent tax laws is recommended), greater control over personal income, and independence from bureaucracy. Usually, independent contractors receive greater gross pay (hourly or per visit rate) than employees because independent contractors are responsible for providing their own benefits, equipment, insurance, and tax withholding.

When practitioners work as employees, the employer may provide health insurance; withhold taxes; provide vacation, sick, and personal leave days; supply equipment and forms; and furnish liability and workers' compensation insurance, and possibly a retirement plan.

Traditionally, speech-language pathology services were furnished on a cost basis. However, since March 1, 1998, speech-language pathology services are reimbursed under salary equivalency rates. Clinicians are urged to see the rates published in the *Federal Register* in order to negotiate a fair and equitable per visit rate plus mileage.

This book uses the independent contractor agreement as the basis of discussions of business practices.

PROGRAM ADMINISTRATION

There are many texts and references regarding the establishment and maintenance of a clinical practice in speech-language pathology. Clinicians who are interested in establishing a private practice in the home health care environment should search out and reference these texts. In addition, it is suggested that clinicians get a solid knowledge base in basic accounting and business practices.

Speech-language pathologists working in home health care as independent practitioners will encounter many program administrative problems similar to those confronting any speech-language pathologist in private practice. Whether directly salaried by the agency or working on some type of a percentage basis or pay per visit rate, speech-language pathologists are expected to organize their portion of the program in an efficient, businesslike manner that will be an asset to the overall program.

The home health agency that enters into an agreement with a speech-language pathologist expects to make a reasonable return on its investment while at the same time seeing significant improvement in the care of the agency's patients who exhibit communication disorders.

The effectiveness of a private speech-language pathologist practice in home health care is determined, to a great extent, by the efficiency of the program procedures. In today's complex home health environment—which includes the existence of national health insurance plans, decreasing Medicare and Medicaid coverage, and an increasing number of private managed care companies and managed Medicare companies—agencies emphasize the necessity for speech-language pathologists to keep up-to-date on all federal regulations relating to Medicare Conditions of Participation, all changes in criteria for reimbursement, and all documentation requirements.

In reference to program coordination, scheduling practices, and referrals made to speech-language pathologists, each agency is highly individual and procedures are usually agency specific. Taking this point into consideration, it would be wise for practicing speech-language pathologists to spend the time to learn about the operations of the agencies that they deal with. In general, however, the speech-language pathologist should be responsible for the following basic program coordination procedures:

- When a patient is released to the care of the speech-language pathologist, or the speech-language pathologist is the only home health service in the home, it is the speech-language pathologist's responsibility to keep other team members informed regarding progress or the appearance of any other problems.
- It is imperative that the speech-language pathologist constantly update his or her skills in the areas of clinical medical rehabilitation, current nursing practices, and diseases and pathogenesis of diseases in patients cared for in the home.
- Speech-language pathologists are responsible for keeping accurate records of visits and charges on the appropriate form for each of the agencies with which they contract. In most instances, the home health agency will have a daily visit record (Exhibit 6–1) from which the posting of charges can be made.
- To minimize patient scheduling problems, for example, insufficient time being scheduled for a particular patient, the clinician should establish a system-

Exhibit 6–1 Daily Visit Report

Therapist: _____
Agency: _____
Date: _____
Discipline: _____

Patient Name / Patient Signature	Patient Number	Service Code	Payer	Discipline Tx or Eval	Quantity	Visit Time	Patient Contact Hrs. Min.
						S F	
						S F	
						S F	
						S F	
						S F	

continues

Exhibit 6–1 continued

S						
F						
S						
F						
S						
F						
S						
F						
S						
F						

Service Codes:

Chargeable: 020 RPT   030 SLP   040 OTR

Nonchargeable: 116 Canceled Visit   117 In Hospital   118 Refused Care   119 Not Home/Not Found

Visit Count:

Chargeable   _____

Nonchargeable   _____

Total   _____

Mileage: End   _____

Begin   _____

Total   _____

I certify that the above information is true and correct.

atic procedure that the home health agency can follow in making referrals. At a minimum, the following information should be included in any type of referral: date of request, start of care, identification information, referral source, services needed, description of the problem, referring or attending physician, and current medications.

REIMBURSEMENT

The information presented in this section is meant to provide speech-language pathologists with a broad overview of reimbursement issues and practices in the home health arena so that they may understand the differences among the various kinds of coverage plans. It is not intended to reflect any of the most recent changes or regulatory differences among different states, intermediaries, or insurance companies.

Speech-language pathologists are advised to confer with the home health agency, intermediary, or third-party payer to confirm the precise provisions for reimbursement for any particular plan or individual. The criteria for coverage and the limitations on services vary depending on the type of insurance plan and/or the individual policy. For example, private payers may limit the number of visits allowed within a specified time frame, whereas Medicare bases the need for continuation of service on continuing functional change.

A clear understanding of the guidelines for reimbursement of speech-language pathology provided in the home will assist clinicians in their effort to provide quality home care to individuals. Reimbursement guidelines may influence treatment by setting parameters for the length and/or type of services that will be covered. When the practitioner is aware of these parameters, decisions abut treatment goals and services can be selected to best serve the patient within the limits allowed. Also, an awareness of reimbursement guidelines can assist practitioners in maintaining a positive relationship with third-party payers and fiscal intermediaries. Given the profession's continuing efforts to improve patients' and administrative personnel's awareness of speech-language pathology, practitioners can more adequately discuss changes in reimbursement patterns as they affect the profession and the home health benefit as a whole. Speech-language pathologists are encouraged to have a broad-based knowledge of reimbursement principles, regardless of the specific payer, as well as specific information about individual payer parameters for reimbursement. With such a background, practitioners can adjust to changes in coverage requirements with relative ease and minimize disruption of their practice and the services they provide to patients.

Although home health services are a benefit provided in a variety of insurance plans, Medicare—the federal government's health insurance plan for Social Security recipients over the age of 65 and persons who are disabled—is by far the primary reimbursement source for home health services in the United States today. Familiarity with the Medicare rules and regulations is helpful because many other plans are patterned after the Medicare system and often follow its lead.

Medicare

The federal government provides home care or funding for such care under a variety of programs created by the Social Security Act, including Medicare (Social Security Act, Title XVIII), Medicaid (Social Security Act, Title XIX), and the Older Americans Act (PL 89-73, 1965; PL 98-459), to name a few. These programs provide specific approaches and funding for specific aspects of home care (Harris, 1997).

Medicare was enacted in July 1965 and became effective on what has since become known as *"M" Day,* July 1, 1966. Medicare is a two-part program commonly referred to as *Medicare Part A* and *Medicare Part B*. Under Medicare Part A, beneficiaries receive certain insurance coverage for hospitalization, specifically defined medical care provided in a skilled nursing facility, and specifically defined home health care. In addition to Part A coverage, Medicare beneficiaries may purchase, for a small monthly premium, supplemental insurance for Part B coverage. Physician services provided on an outpatient basis, home health care, pathology services, outpatient hospital services, and other services are covered by Part B. Part B services are defined in terms of the specifics involved and may be furnished by individuals such as physicians, medical supply providers, and therapists. As of July 1, 1981, Part A actually pays for home health services to beneficiaries who are covered by both Part A and Part B (*Home Health and Hospice Manual,* Section 203.3). Coverage under Part A is summarized in Table 6–1.

Medicare Part A and Part B differ in the way that they are billed and reimbursed. Institutional or individual providers must use different procedures and forms in billing for Medicare Part A and Part B. Under Part A, Medicare will reimburse the provider 100 percent of the allowable charge, but under Part B it will reimburse only 80 percent of the allowable charge. The remaining 20 percent must be billed to the individual patient or to the patient's supplementary insurance plan.

Although home health is a reimbursable service under both Medicare Part A and Part B, because of the differences in billing procedures and reimbursement formulas, most home health agencies do not choose to bill under both plans. The majority of agencies bill primarily under Part A. Individual occupational therapists working in their own private practice and who are certified as Medicare Part B providers may bill under Part B but must follow all required billing and reimbursement procedures and will need to bill both Medicare and the patient.

In addition to skilled nursing and home health aide services, covered home health care services are physical therapy, occupational therapy, and speech therapy. Occupational therapy helps beneficiaries gain the necessary skills to per-

Table 6-1 Speech-Language Pathology Treatment Guidelines under Medicare Part A

Treatment Guide	Dysarthria without Aphasia	Laryngectomy	Glossectomy	Dysphagia Due to Surgical Deficit
Periodically not covered	Patient not sufficiently alert to be evaluated.	Patient cannot follow directions or has severe comprehension difficulties.	Patient cannot follow directions.	Deficit is so severe as to preclude any possibility of swallowing.
Evaluation with 1–3 visits	Patient cannot follow directions. Mild deficits. Home education program established.	Evaluation could include 1 session preop as outpatient.		Mild deficits not needing over 3 visits.
Evaluation and maintenance program with 1–3 visits	Many patients with pure dysarthria may continue oral-motor strengthening exercises that do not require skilled intervention.		Patient's family to monitor exercises with periodic reevaluation; total glossectomy.	Patient severity low enough that instructions to patient, family are sufficient. Almost 25% of patients will fall within this category.
Under 2 weeks	Patients with progressive	Many patients are seen 3× weekly during the initial week.	Severity so great as to preclude oral	

continues

Table 6–1 continued

Treatment Guide	Dysarthria without Aphasia	Laryngectomy	Glossectomy	Dysphagia Due to Surgical Deficit
	neurological diseases like Parkinson's who need neuromuscular reeducation to maintain current level of functioning.		speech potential and augmentative communication device is recommended (treatment may resume for 1–5 visits when device is obtained).	
Under 1 month		Most patients are seen no more than 2 to 3 times per week after the first month.		
Under 2 months	Most dysarthric patients without aphasia finished with treatment by 2 months postonset.	Most patients with tracheoesophageal puncture (TEP) prostheses—typically under 20 visits total. Most patients without TEP are seen no more than 2× per week after the second month.	Most patients are finished with treatment.	Most patients finished with treatment under 2 months postonset.

continues

Table 6–1 continued

Treatment Guide	Dysarthria without Aphasia	Laryngectomy	Glossectomy	Dysphagia Due to Surgical Deficit
Under 4 months		Most patients are finished with treatment by 4 months postonset. Those patients who continue in treatment after the 4 months are seen less than once a week.		
Under 6 months		Patient may have had radiation or chemotherapy treatments necessitating a period of no treatments.		
Under 12 months				
Reason for evaluation and therapy when onset has been too long	No previous treatment; new technology becomes available.	No previous treatment; new technology becomes available.	No previous treatment; new technology becomes available.	No previous treatment; new technology becomes available.

continues

Table 6–1 continued

Treatment Guide	Aphasia	Dysphagia Due to Neuromotor Deficit	Nonhemispheric Disorder (linguistic-pragmatic-orientation-memory)
Periodically not covered	Patient is not sufficiently alert to be evaluated.	Patient not medically stable enough for evaluation.	Patient unable to respond, not sufficiently alert.
Evaluation with 1–3 visits	Aphasia due to transient ischemic attacks. Degree of severity of aphasia is so great as to constitute no realistic progress. Severity of deficit not great enough to warrant treatment.	Patient not a candidate for swallowing, or patient's swallowing adequate for present diet.	Patient rejects treatment.
Evaluation and maintenance program with 1–3 visits	Degree of severity too severe to warrant intervention; however, clinician can train family and/or caregivers in patient's maintenance program.	Develop teaching swallow precautions to family, patient, and caregivers.	
Under 2 weeks	Evaluation indicates that progress may be possible and clinician attempts trial treatment, which proves nonproductive plateau and reached goals.		
Under 1 month			

continues

Table 6–1 continued

Treatment Guide	Aphasia	Dysphagia Due to Neuromotor Deficit	Nonhemispheric Disorder (linguistic-pragmatic-orientation-memory)
Under 2 months		Most patients are finished with treatment in 2 months postonset.	
Under 4 months	Most aphasic patients are finished with treatment by 4 months postonset.		Most patients finished under 3 months.
Under 6 months	Continues to show significant progress toward stated and functional goals. Patient's functional communicative improvement continues to impact significantly on quality of life. Almost all patients will be finished with treatment by 6 months.		Continues to show significant progress toward stated goals and functional outcomes.
Under 12 months	Patient will be returning to normal capabilities. Very few patients continue in treatment up to 12 months. Treatment has been unavailable on a consistent basis.		
Reason for evaluation and therapy when onset has been too long	No previous treatment. Has good rehab potential.	No previous treatment.	No previous treatment.

Source: Reprinted from *Region 5 Edit Guidelines*, Health Care Financing Administration.

form the activities of daily living, while physical therapy helps patients regain physical functional skills, such as increased mobility. Speech therapy is provided to help patients overcome speech, language, and swallowing problems related to the physical condition that required home care. For any of the services covered by Medicare, there must be a general restorative potential demonstrated in the treatment of the patient (*Home Health and Hospice Manual,* Section 205). Several visits would be allowed to teach a patient how to maintain function if there is no restorative potential. Although physical therapy, occupational therapy, and speech therapy are services that can be rendered either at the patient's home or in a hospital outpatient department, skilled nursing facility, or rehab center, only when the services are actually rendered at a patient's home will they be reimbursed under Medicare's home care provision.

In general, to receive any of the services, Medicare beneficiaries must meet program requirements. They must, for example, be homebound (*1986 Medicare Explained,* Section 420.63). To be considered homebound, patients must have physical impairments making access to outside care difficult. Patients need not be bedridden, however. Lack of readily available transportation does not constitute a homebound status. The program also requires that the patient be under the care of a physician. Further qualifications for home health care are discussed later in this chapter.

Documentation is one of the biggest challenges of working in the home health care arena. Unlike most traditional speech-language pathology work settings where documentation may consist of a few lines for each visit, home health agency guidelines require daily set notes that reflect the movement toward short-term or long-term goals and show improvement in the patient's overall communicative ability. In addition to detailed daily progress notes, the clinician must complete a progress-to-date note on a monthly basis showing progress and detailed treatment for each month. Each patient is also recertified by his or her physician every 60 days, at which time the patient must be reevaluated, treatment goals revised or added, and justification for continued treatment documented.

Although there are many methods of reimbursement under Medicare, they are not detailed herein. Anyone providing home health care services should be familiar with reimbursement principles, and clinicians are encouraged to read the HIM-11 (*Health Insurance Manual-11*) provided by the Health Care Financing Administration (HCFA). To the independent contractor, methods of reimbursement are usually not that significant, but reimbursement is necessary to ensure a financially stable program. Independent practitioners should be familiar with basic tenets of Medicare reimbursement.

Under the Medicare program, there are three methods of determining reimbursement to providers:

144 THE SPEECH-LANGUAGE PATHOLOGIST IN HOME HEALTH CARE

1. reasonable costs
2. reasonable charge
3. prospective payment

Home health agencies are reimbursed under the reasonable cost method, that is, on the basis of the cost deemed necessary to deliver services efficiently to beneficiaries. Each method takes into consideration both direct and indirect costs. To determine reasonable costs, the HCFA carries out a process called *cost finding,* which is facilitated by the home health agencies' completing the Cost Report (HCFA Form 1728).

Cost Limits

Cost limits are the predetermined maximums placed on per visit reimbursable costs, by discipline, to ensure the efficient delivery of care (Harris, 1994). Section 223 of the Social Security Amendments of 1972 granted the authority for limits to be set on the costs that Medicare would recognize as reasonable through the overall efficient delivery of home health care services. Cost limits are developed using local and nonlocal costs as separate costs. Before June 5, 1985, the per discipline limits were established by type of service and compared with the per discipline costs in the aggregate based on the number of visits for each type of service. The aggregate was used to determine if the home health agency was above the limit. Starting on July 1, 1985, the limit was issued, and its impact calculated by the individual disciplines (Commerce Clearinghouse, 1986).

Each year the *Federal Register* sets forth the new schedule of limits on home health agency costs. Although the goal is to establish cost limits based on the actual costs in the industry, there has been a problem in obtaining reliable information on a current basis.

The significance to independent contractors is the fact that their charges to the home health agency are capitated. Speech-language pathologists must know the cost limits as issued by the federal government in order to adequately negotiate a fair and equitable price for services. Information from the *Federal Register* is available in publications from the HCFA, in numerous home health publications, and now on the Internet.

Specific Guidelines

For a patient to receive home health benefits under either Part A or Part B, prior hospitalization is not required. The number of home health visits is not limited arbitrarily but depends on the beneficiary's progress. Intermediaries issue guidelines about visit frequencies; however, the guidelines are not meant to be restrictive.

The HCFA has established federal regulations for the Medicare system. The actual administration of the program and interpretation of the regulations are carried out by a designated fiscal intermediary, that is, an insurance company chosen to represent Medicare. All home health agencies are assigned to one of 10 regional intermediaries who have contracted with the government to carry out Medicare's business in a designated region. Significantly, intermediaries may differ in their interpretations and enforcement of HCFA guidelines. For instance, what is accepted intermediary practice in California may not be accepted intermediary practice in Texas. Consequently, clinicians should be familiar with their own intermediary's guidelines and interpretations.

Eligibility Criteria. To be eligible for Part A home health benefits under Medicare, the patient must

- *Be homebound.* The patient does not have to be bedridden and may even leave the home, on infrequent occasions, such as for a physician's appointment. In general, homebound means that to leave the home requires a considerable and taxing effort on the patient's part and requires the assistance of another person or a device.
- *Have a physician referral.* The patient must be under the care of a physician who certifies that home health services are indicated.
- *Require skilled services.* The patient is initially in need of physical therapy, speech-language pathology, or skilled nursing services on an intermittent basis.

Patients are eligible to receive home health benefits as long as the preceding criteria are met.

Criteria for Speech-Language Pathology Coverage. The need for speech-language pathology services does qualify a patient for Part A benefits, as does the need for nursing or physical therapy (Appendix 6–A). This means that a patient can qualify (after meeting the eligibility requirements) for Part A home health benefits solely on the basis of communication/cognition/swallowing deficits. This can be a great advantage to the speech-language pathologist; however, it is also the duty of the speech-language pathologist to document how the communication disorder makes the patient homebound, especially if no physical disabilities exist.

Other criteria that must be met for speech-language pathology to be covered are as follows:

- There must be a specific physician's order for speech-language pathology.
- Treatment must be performed by a qualified speech-language pathologist.

- Treatment must be reasonable and necessary for the patient's illness or injury.

The term *reasonable and necessary* is open to interpretation. Medicare does not define this term specifically. Understanding how Medicare defines this term can be helpful to the clinician because decisions about reimbursement and payment may be based on misinterpretation. For this reason, it is very important that clinicians be able to predict outcomes and that they document very carefully any contraindications to treatment or any aberrations of the patient or family that could influence or delay the expected outcome in the time frame predicted. In addition, the effects of the new prospective payment system are unclear at this point, but changes certainly will occur. Exhibit 6–2 presents guidelines from the HCFA that clinicians should consider in determining whether their treatment is reasonable and necessary.

Review of Service/Denial of Payment. Periodically during the treatment process, Medicare's designated intermediary (a financial and medical review board assigned to a specific region of the country) reviews the appropriateness of the frequency of visits, the date of onset, and the documented progress. The reviewers are generally nurses, who may or may not be familiar with speech-language pathology. Thus, the quality of visit-related documentation plays a very important role in obtaining reimbursement. Good documentation demonstrates the progress necessary for reimbursement, and it also serves as justification for continued treatment or the termination of care. Medicare intermediaries look for significant practical and functional improvement that is well paced over a reasonable period. Denials of Medicare coverage occur in the following circumstances:

- Eligibility criteria are not met; for example, the patient is not homebound, there are no physician orders, and/or the need for intermittent physical therapy, speech-language pathology, or skilled nursing is not evident.
- The need for the speech-language pathologist's skilled service is not reasonable or necessary.
- Significant progress has not been documented.
- Duplication of services exists.
- Fraud or abuse of program policies occurs.

Practitioners should realize that denial can always be appealed when a reasonable justification that is consistent with Medicare guidelines exists. Medicare provides for a formal appeals process that home health agencies may use. Practitioners are encouraged to pursue this process and participate when warranted. They

Exhibit 6–2 General Principles Governing Reasonable and Necessary Services

1. The service of a physical, a speech-language pathology, or an occupational thera-pist is a skilled therapy service if the inherent complexity of the service is such that it can be performed safely and/or effectively only by or under the general supervision of a skilled therapist. To be covered, the skilled services must also be reasonable and necessary to the treatment of the patient's illness or injury or to the restoration or maintenance of function affected by the patient's illness or in-jury. It is necessary to determine whether individual therapy services are skilled and whether, in view of the patient's overall condition, skilled management of the services provided is needed although many or all of the specific services needed to treat the illness or injury do not require the skills of a therapist.

2. The development, implementation, management, and evaluation of a patient care plan based on the physician's orders constitute skilled therapy services when, because of the patient's condition, those activities required the involvement of a skilled therapist to meet the patient's needs, promote recovery, and ensure medi-cal safety. Where the skills of a therapist are needed to manage and periodically reevaluate the appropriateness of a maintenance program because of an identified danger to the patient, such services would be covered even if the skills of a thera-pist are not needed to carry out the activities performed as part of the maintenance program.

3. While a patient's particular medical condition is a valid factor in deciding if skilled therapy services are needed, the diagnosis or prognosis should never be the sole factor in deciding that a service is or is not skilled. The key issue is whether the skills of a therapist are needed to treat the illness or injury, or whether the services can be carried out by nonskilled personnel.

4. A service that is ordinarily considered nonskilled could be considered a skilled therapy service in cases in which there is clear documentation that, because of special medical complications, skilled rehabilitation personnel are required to perform or supervise the service or to observe the patient; however, the impor-tance of a particular service to a patient or the frequency with which it must be performed does not, by itself, make nonskilled service a skilled service.

5. The skilled therapy services must be reasonable and necessary to the treatment of the patient's illness or injury within the context of the patient's unique medical condition. To be considered reasonable and necessary for the treatment of the illness or injury:

   a. The services must be consistent with the nature and severity of the illness or injury and the patient's particular medical needs, including the requirement that the amount, frequency, and duration of the services must be reasonable.

   b. The services must be considered, under accepted standards of medical prac-tice, to be specific, safe, and effective treatment for the patient's condition; and

continues

Exhibit 6–2 continued

> c. The services must be provided with the expectation, based on the assessment made by the physician of the patient's rehabilitation potential, that:
>   1) The condition of the patient will improve materially in a reasonable and generally predictable period of time; or
>   2) The services are necessary to the establishment of a safe and effective maintenance program.
>
>   Services involving activities for the general welfare of any patient, e.g., general exercises to promote overall fitness or flexibility and activities to provide diversion or general motivation, do not constitute skilled therapy. Those services can be performed by nonskilled individuals without the supervision of a therapist.
>
> d. Services of skilled therapists for the purpose of teaching the patient, family, or caregivers necessary techniques, exercises, or precautions are covered to the extent that they are reasonable and necessary to treat illness or injury; however, visits made by skilled therapists to a patient's home solely to train other home health agency (HHA) staff, e.g., home health aides, are not billable as visits since the HHA is responsible for ensuring that its staff are properly trained to perform any service it furnishes. The cost of a skilled therapist's visit for the purpose of training HHA staff is an administrative cost to the agency.
>
> e. The amount, frequency, and duration of the services must be reasonable.
>
> **EXAMPLE**
>   A patient with a diagnosis of multiple sclerosis has recently been discharged from the hospital following an exacerbation of her condition that has left her wheelchair bound and, for the first time, without any expectation of achieving ambulation again. The physician has ordered physical therapy to select the proper wheelchair for her long-term use and to teach safe use of the wheelchair and safe transfer techniques to the patient and family. Physical therapy would be reasonable and necessary to evaluate the patient's overall needs, to make the selection of the proper wheelchair, and to teach the patient and family safe use of the wheelchair and proper transfer techniques.
>
> *Source:* Adapted from Health Care Financing Administration.

should check with the agency regarding the exact procedure. It is not uncommon for denials to be reversed when further information is presented and careful review of documentation is conducted.

Medicaid

Medicaid is a federally regulated, state-administered program. Its purpose is to provide health care to the poor and medically indigent. The cost of the program is shared by the state and federal government. The 1967 Social Security Amendments, which went into effect in 1970, require most states to provide home health coverage to Medicaid beneficiaries who are also eligible for care in a skilled nursing facility. Coverage varies from state to state because under Medicaid, occupational therapy is considered an optional service. Medicaid differs from Medicare in that qualifying skilled services (nursing and physical therapy) are not necessarily prerequisites for speech-language therapy and the patient may not always need to be homebound (Trossman, 1984). However, this interpretation varies from state to state, so the regulation in a particular state should be checked.

Overall, limits on Medicaid reimbursement rates are significantly lower than Medicare reimbursement limits, and increasing numbers of agencies are turning away Medicaid recipients. A few states allow therapists to receive individual Medicaid provider numbers. These therapists can accept assignments and bill Medicaid directly for therapy in the home. Current eligibility for a Medicaid benefit period should be checked before services begin, because prior authorization to start services can vary dramatically, slowing the initiation of treatment.

Home health agencies that wish to provide services to Medicaid recipients must demonstrate certification under Medicare before submitting any charges. Patients covered by both Medicare and Medicaid who receive home health services are expected to sign the appropriate forms so that the agency can submit claims to Medicare first and then file additional claims with Medicaid. Most Medicaid programs require that services be rendered in a patient's own residence, or that of a relative, and that a plan of care be established by the patient's attending physician.

Private Insurance

Benefits for speech-language pathology under private health insurance plans vary greatly. Most basic hospital and major medical policies provide benefits for inpatient hospital occupational therapy services; however, speech-language pathology services are not a diagnosis-related group (DRG) covered service. Coverage for outpatient or home health services is less uniform. Generally, policies either specify speech-language pathology as a covered service or it is not specifically mentioned. Rarely is speech-language pathology named as being excluded; however, when speech-language pathology services are not specifically named, it is advisable to check with the insurer and explain the services to be offered. Often, such action will result in appropriate coverage.

Private insurance plans are more likely than Medicare to place limits on the frequency and duration of therapy visits as well as on the amount that will be paid. Some policies require a copayment from the insured to assist with costs.

It is important to remember that benefits must be confirmed policy by policy. That is, two patients with the same insurance carrier and with levels of insurance benefits that appear to be similar may actually have different access to services. Because of this lack of consistency in coverage within and between companies, the type of benefits available is usually investigated by the home health agency before it accepts a referral.

Managed Care Plans

Managed care plans are an alternative to the traditional model of insurance service delivery. They were originally mandated by Congress in the 1970s and were designed to govern care in a way that would decrease costs. They have grown dramatically, and a large proportion of the population is currently insured under some form of a managed care plan.

One of the most popular forms of managed care plans is the health maintenance organization (HMO). HMOs provide a comprehensive range of services to their members. Members pay a fixed premium at regular intervals and receive needed health care services without any additional costs or with only a small copayment. To remain successful and retain their ability to attract and keep members, and to remain profitable, HMOs must provide needed services to satisfy their members, yet not overuse services and threaten their profitability. Most HMOs provide a basic home health benefit that covers the traditional Medicare home health services such as nursing and physical therapy.

Speech-language pathology may or may not be included in the HMO plans available in a given area. HMOs that service Medicare beneficiaries (called *federally qualified HMOs*) must provide all of the benefits Medicare provides, including speech-language pathology. The need to produce a positive financial outcome will often dictate the decision regarding how many therapy visits may be provided in any HMO plan. Practitioners can influence this decision by becoming aware of who makes the decision about the service delivery in the HMO and by clearly articulating the positive patient outcomes and resulting financial savings provided by speech-language therapy interventions.

When speech-language pathology is covered as a benefit, limitations on the number of home health visits are often set. Coordination among disciplines becomes important when the HMO limits total home health visits. Disciplines must decide the most advantageous way to divide services and achieve the best patient outcome.

The preferred provider organization (PPO) is a form of managed care that is a blend of a private pay plan and an HMO. It is an arrangement for service delivery. Members of a PPO pay a set premium, but their choice of service providers, although broader than that in an HMO, is more restricted than in a purely private plan, and often an additional copayment for service is required. Service providers are designated as "preferred" and consist of groups or individuals with whom the PPO has negotiated set and agreed-upon fees that are often discounted (Scott &

Somers, 1997). "Nonpreferred" providers may be used by PPO members, but the member must pay the higher proportion of the costs. A home health agency may be a designated provider in a PPO.

Most PPOs offer home health benefits. Provision of a home health benefit in a PPO varies. As with an HMO, preauthorization and limitations on the number of visits are very common when home health is covered by a PPO.

Department of Veterans Affairs

Although not a major reimbursement source for most home health agencies, the Department of Veterans Affairs (VA) reimburses providers for certain home health services if specific qualifying conditions are fulfilled. The patient must be homebound, and services must be ordered by a physician. The condition to be treated may be either a service-related condition, for example, diabetes that developed during the veteran's active duty and was treated at that time, or a nonservice-connected condition that has been reviewed by a rating board to determine the veteran's eligibility for the Aid and Attendance Homebound Program. Reimbursement from the VA is contingent on prior approval in the latter case, which is obtained from VA regional offices and not directly from the VA hospital.

Federal Employee's Blue Cross/Blue Shield

The Federal Employee's Blue Cross/Blue Shield plan offers both a high option and a standard option to its members. The high option provides more extensive coverage than that of the standard option with lower deductibles and copayments for the insured. Speech-language pathology is covered under both options on an outpatient basis but is covered on a home health basis only under the high option plan. The therapy that is provided must be part of an approved home health care program.

Business Ethics in Reimbursement

As the demand for health care services has grown and reimbursement has become more available, the competition for the reimbursement dollar has increased. As a result, service providers have become more sensitive to the bottom line, and reimbursement issues often assume a central role in decision making and planning. The pressures to maximize reimbursement are felt in all arenas of practice and appear to be intensifying. In the home health setting, these pressures can be problematic for the speech-language pathologist.

Practitioners in home health need to be sensitive to the reimbursement pressures that can influence their practice and be aware of the ethical and legal problems these pressures may present. Fraud and abuse in reimbursement can occur in many ways, but perhaps the most common problems in home health are billing the insurer for treatment that was not actually provided and providing very brief or minimal service while seeking full reimbursement. These practices can occur more easily in home health than in some other settings as a result of the isolated nature of home health services delivery. Therapy providers see patients alone, and other agency representatives are not available to verify whether services were actually provided or how long they lasted. The fact that service providers may be working on a contractual basis in which their income depends on the number of visits they complete can provide a tempting opportunity for some practitioners to "pad" the number of visits they perform in order to increase their income. General productivity standards that target a particular number of visits that employees are expected to complete can also pressure practitioners, who may be behind in their work, to document treatment visits that may not have occurred.

Each of these situations presents the practitioner with an ethical decision. Individuals practicing in home health should be alert to the possibility of experiencing conflicting pressures and values and must understand how to address them. Awareness of possible problems in this area can enable practitioners to recognize problems when they occur and assist them in avoiding fraudulent and abusive practices. Practitioners also need to be alert to what is occurring around them. Each individual has a professional and an ethical responsibility to report fraud and abuse when they are identified or observed. Efforts to bring the problem to the attention of the individuals involved and their supervisors should occur first. If the problems are not remedied, abuse should be reported to higher authorities. Medicare, for example, maintains a 24-hour fraud and abuse hotline (800-368-5779) that can be used to report violations.

MARKETING

One of the most difficult aspects of independent home health contracting is that of marketing. Most speech-language pathologists have no experience in this area and seem to be at a loss when trying to identify potential contacts. Information is available from the American Speech-Language-Hearing Association, which provides several workshops and printed materials on the marketing aspects of a speech-language pathology practice. This section presents some marketing techniques that have proven effective in closing a contract.

Developing Contacts

"Where to begin?" is a question frequently asked. The first step in marketing is to find leads, which can be done in several ways. The Yellow Pages can provide a wealth of information about area agencies and the types of services they provide.

Also, the practitioner should contact the state planning authority or the agency that governs health care in his or her state. Most states have a roster of facilities listed by type, such as hospitals, nursing homes, and home health agencies. Again, this roster can provide valuable information for marketing. Finally, the clinician is always read the want ads in the local paper. Agencies often advertise positions, and the practitioner can find leads.

After establishing some leads, the practitioner uses the marketing strategies of cold calling, networking, and participating in the community. Figure 6–1 shows the marketing paradigm that can be used when the clinician is marketing home health care agencies. Exhibit 6–3 lists techniques the clinician can use for the marketing strategies of cold calling, networking, and community participation.

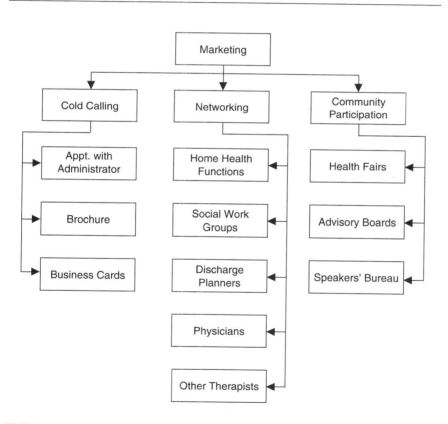

FIGURE 6–1 Home Health Care Marketing Paradigm. *Source:* Copyright © 1997, Cecil G. Betros, Jr.

Exhibit 6–3 Marketing Techniques

COLD CALLING
1. If possible, try to talk to the administrator or the director of nursing.
2. Always tell the receptionist the purpose of the call and the time needed.
3. If you are turned down, do the following:
   • Send a follow-up letter, enclosing your business card.
   • Call again in six months.
4. If you get an appointment:
   • Take a brochure and/or résumé.
   • Dress professionally.
   • Always have a business card.
   • Bring a short summary of your qualifications and services.
5. Try to find out what speech-language pathology services the agency makes available, if any, and who is providing the services.
6. Find out what aspects of the current speech-language pathology service the administrator likes and does not like.
7. Show how you can improve the current provision of services.
8. Always be prepared to offer some "giveaways," for example:
   • free inservice for one year
   • no charge for continuous quality improvement activities
   • no charge for staff meetings
9. If the person is hesitant to change or to add you to the contractor list, always ask for a trial to prove yourself.
10. Never promise something you cannot deliver.
11. Market any techniques you have developed that improve patient care or improve the staff competencies.
12. Show the administrator any outcome data you may have.

NETWORKING
1. Attend state and local home health functions.
2. Be sure you are on all local home health mailing lists.
3. Belong to at least one home health organization.
4. Make it known to the local home health agencies that you are available for inservices for their staffs.
5. Present at local social work/discharge planner functions in your city.
6. Network with physicians who refer to a particular agency.
   • Make visits to their office or take them to lunch.
   • Remember, all it takes is one good case for a physician to use your services.
   • Ask physicians to specifically request your services from the home health agency.

continues

Exhibit 6–3 continued

> **COMMUNITY PARTICIPATION**
> 1. Participate in community health fairs and exhibits.
> 2. Participate in the home health advisory boards.
> 3. Get your name on a health care speakers' bureau.

Contracting and Negotiating

Another difficult area for the independent contractor in speech-language pathology is negotiating a professional services contract. The clinician's success at negotiating a contract depends on four major factors, as depicted in Figure 6–2. These factors are competition, supply, demand, and capitation and reimbursement of fees.

Clinicians must know the competition so that they can determine what types of services to provide and what fees to charge. Also very critical to competition is knowing the demographic areas that the competition covers. In gathering data on the competition, clinicians should always behave in a professional manner and never speak negatively about competitors to an administrator. At times an administrator may make negative comments about the agency's current contractor, in

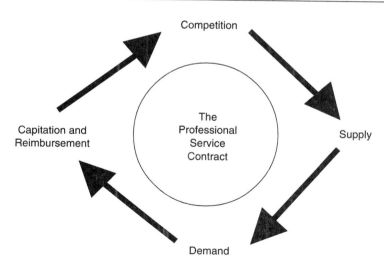

Figure 6–2 Contract Negotiation Paradigm. *Source:* Copyright © 1998, Cecil G. Betros, Jr.

which case a good policy is to nod, indicating understanding, and then to continue with the negotiating process.

Supply also has a great impact on the type of contract that the clinician can negotiate. Obviously, in large metropolitan areas where there might be a sufficient supply of speech-language pathologists doing home health care, clinicians might be less likely to negotiate a contract, or they might not be able to charge the fees that they had anticipated because of the overabundance of clinicians in the area. Conversely, in more rural areas where there is a lack of speech-language pathology services, clinicians may have more flexibility in the private contract and the fees that they can charge.

Some administrators fail to see the demand for speech-language pathology services in home health care. An administrator may say, "We have only one or two patients who use it. I don't see the need to contract for the service." In this case, the clinician must increase the administrator's awareness of demand that most likely does exist. One key way to do this is to make the administrator aware of the types of speech-language pathology referrals that may be obtained. The administrator may point to the agency's low percentage of patients with strokes. The clinician then needs to explain the cognitive-linguistic problems associated with all types of diseases, how speech-language pathology services fit into the continuum of medical care, and where the speech-language pathologist can fit into this continuum. Speech-language pathologists often have to create the demand for their services. This can be done easily by presenting a few inservices for staff nurses, home health aides, and other therapists.

It is imperative that the speech-language pathologist know and understand capitation amounts (maximum allowable charges) and reimbursement issues that influence speech-language pathology services and home health. Clinicians should know the amount of allowable charges under the Medicare system for home health agencies in their particular area, as well as the usual and customary charges from other clinicians in the area, to come up with a final figure for home care services.

A clinician who does not know the actual costs of delivering services may make a fatal mistake in contract negotiation. Clinicians should never sign a contract just to get a contract, but should sit down and analyze the cost per visit. Clinicians should ask the administrator about the agency's current and expected volume of speech-language pathology services. The greater the volume, the lower the cost will be per visit, which means the clinician can offer a better rate to the agency. Also, it is important for the practitioner to keep in mind the amount of time needed to drive from one house to another when he or she is calculating fees.

As their independent practice begins to grow, clinicians often wonder when they should hire another practitioner. A good rule of thumb is to hire when there is enough work for a half-time clinician. That is usually the break-even point for the self-employed clinician.

Exhibit 6–4 outlines the elements that a contract should have. Appendix 6–A is an example of a fee-for-service contract. Although contracts are written in many forms, this example is provided to show the typical wording and construction of a contract.

Exhibit 6–4 Rehabilitation Therapy Services Agreement

    I. Background Information
   II. Agreement
       A. Services
       B. Documentation and Records
       C. Coordination of Services
  III. Compensation and Billing
       A. Compensation
       B. Billing
       C. Reimbursement Denial
   IV. Representations and Warranties
       A. Provider Representations and Warranties
       B. Agency Representations and Warranties
    V. Indemnification
   VI. Insurance
  VII. Term and Termination of Agreement
       A. Term
       B. Termination
          1. Termination without Cause
          2. Termination for Breach
          3. Termination Due to Loss of License
          4. Termination Due to Legislative or Administrative Change
          5. Effect of Termination
 VIII. Confidentiality
       A. Information
       B. Terms of This Agreement
       C. Patient Information
   IX. Independent Contractor
    X. Access to Records
   XI. Civil Rights
  XII. Miscellaneous
       A. Alternative Dispute Resolution
       B. *Force Majeure*
       C. Entire Agreement: Modification

continues

Exhibit 6–4 continued

> D. Applicable Law and Remedies
> E. Notices
> F. Waiver
> G. Captions
> H. Agreement: Binding Effect
> I. Counterparts

CONCLUSION

Speech-language pathologists should confirm the guidelines for reimbursement for speech-language pathology directly with their agency and/or the third-party payer. Lack of coverage or denial of coverage should not be accepted as a final decision. Often, additional contact with the third-party payer and further explanation of the services provided can change the initial decision.

Just as important, speech-language pathologists should keep up-to-date on legislative and regulatory changes that affect the practice of home health. Advocacy and participation in the political process are a necessary function of health care professionals in today's environment. Without an understanding of reimbursement guidelines and legislative or regulatory initiatives, speech-language pathologists will find it very difficult to provide quality care to patients, which is the profession's primary goal. In addition, independent practitioners are expected to operate a well-organized business, using accepted standards of accounting and ethical business practices, and must be able to apply reimbursement principles to the services they provide.

REFERENCES

Commerce Clearinghouse. (1986). *Medicare explained.* Chicago: Author.

Harris, M.D. (1994). *Handbook of home health care administration.* Gaithersburg, MD: Aspen Publishers.

Harris, M.D. (1997). *Handbook of home health care administration* (3rd ed.). Gaithersburg, MD: Aspen Publishers.

Scott, S., & Somers, F. (1997). Payment for occupational therapy services. In J. Blau & M. Gray (Eds.), *The occupational therapy manager.* Rockville, MD: American Occupational Therapy Association.

Trossman, P. (1984). Administrative and professional issues for the occupational therapist in home health care. *American Journal of Occupational Therapy, 38*(11), 726–733.

SUGGESTED READING

Health Care Financing Administration. (1989). *Medicare home health agency manual* (Publication No. HIM-11). Baltimore: Author.

Health Care Financing Administration. (1990). *Medicare intermediary manual,* Part 3, *Claims process* (DHHS Transmittal No. 1487, Section 3906.4). Washington, DC: U.S. Government Printing Office.

Office of the Civilian Health and Medical Program of the Uniformed Services. (1989). *CHAMPUS policy manual* (6010.47-M). Aurora, CO: Author.

Sample Fee-for-Service Rehabilitation Services Agreement

THIS AGREEMENT made this _____ between _____ (hereinafter referred to as "FACILITY") and _____ a provider of Rehabilitation Services, whose address is _____ (hereinafter referred to as "Provider"):

AGREEMENT

1. TERMS

The term of this agreement shall be one (1) year from the date of its execution and shall automatically renew from year to year thereafter unless otherwise terminated as herein provided. Either party hereto may at any time during the term hereof terminate this Agreement upon thirty (30) days' written notice to the other party of such termination. At the end of said thirty (30) days' notice period, this agreement shall forthwith terminate for all purposes, as if said date set forth herein as the termination date of this agreement, provided that any obligations arising prior to the termination of the Agreement shall be governed by the terms hereinafter set forth until satisfied.

2. SERVICES

Rehab services to include Physical Therapy, Occupational Therapy, and Speech-Language Therapy will be furnished in accordance with the plan of care established/certified by the physician responsible for the patient's care.

The service will be performed on the premises of the Facility or in the patient's home and will meet the requirements of Section 1861 (j) (1) of the Social Security Act and of 42 CFR 405.1721 (a).

3. RECORDS

Provider agrees to keep and maintain such records on the services rendered by Provider to patients as may be required by fiscal intermediary; federal, state, or local governmental agency; Facility; or other party to whom billings for Provider's services are rendered. Provider agrees to make all records on Facility's patients to whom Provider has rendered service available for Facility inspection upon request.

4. ADDITIONAL SERVICES

In addition to providing services to patients in the facility, the Provider will advise and participate in the development of Facility's training programs, including staff inservice programs. Provider will act as a consultant to the Facility and will make recommendations to such administration, assist in implementation progress to facilitate compliance by the Facility with all governmental or third-party payer requirements. Written reports will be submitted by Provider as may from time to time be required by Facility.

5. INDEPENDENT CONTRACTOR

It is the party's intention that the Provider shall be an <u>independent contractor and not the Facility's employee.</u> In conformity therewith, the Provider shall retain sole and absolute discretion and judgment in the manner and means of providing services to the Facility. This agreement shall not be construed as a partnership and Facility shall not be liable for any obligations incurred by the Provider. However, Provider shall comply with all policies, rules, and regulations of the Facility in connection with provision of the Provider's services. All service rendered by the Provider shall be rendered in a competent, efficient, and satisfactory manner and in strict accordance with currently approved methods and practices of the Provider's profession.

6. PROVIDER'S QUALIFICATIONS

All services to patients in the Facility shall be performed by Registered Physical Therapist, Licensed Physical Therapy Assistant, Licensed Occupational Therapist, Certified Occupational Therapy Assistant, Speech-Language Pathologists, and Speech-Language Pathologist, CFY, all licensed by the State of _____.

7. INSURANCE

Provider shall procure and maintain professional liability insurance coverage of at least $1,000,000 per occurrence and $3,000,000 annual aggregate. A copy of the Certificate of Insurance evidencing such coverage is available on request. Provider shall indemnify and hold harmless Facility from all costs, expenses, and damages resulting from the negligence of Provider.

8. CIVIL RIGHTS

Provider agrees to comply with Title VI of the Civil Rights Act of 1964 and all requirements imposed by or pursuant to the regulation of the Department of Health, Education and Welfare (45 CFR Prt. 80) issued pursuant to the Title, to the end that, no person in the United States shall, on the ground of race, color, or national origin, be excluded from the participation in, be denied the benefit for which Federal funds are used in support of the Provider's activities.

9. COMPENSATION

Provider will be compensated by Facility for rehabilitation services rendered on a Fee-for-Service basis from the first to the last day of each month (hereinafter referred to as the "billing period") according to invoices submitted to the Facility no later than five (5) working days following the end of the billing period in which said services were rendered. The following fees for service are agreed upon between the parties:

Home Health Patients:
Speech-Language Evaluation	$ _____
Speech-Language Treatment	$ _____
Occupational Therapy Evaluation	$ _____
Occupational Therapy Treatment	$ _____
Certified Occupational Therapy Assistant	$ _____
Physical Therapy Evaluation	$ _____
Physical Therapy Treatment	$ _____
Licensed Physical Therapy Assistant	$ _____
Mileage	$ _____ /mile

A treatment is based on 30 minutes of billable patient services.

Provider's invoices will include the following: (a) the name of the contractor who provided the services, (b) names of patients to whom services were provided and the date(s) and description(s) of services rendered to each patient, (c) the charges applicable to each patient.

Any amendments or changes to the schedule of fees hereinafter stated shall be effective thirty (30) days following the date upon which the parties agree to such amendment or change in writing. Upon the parties' mutual acceptance in writing, the amended schedule of fees shall become part of this agreement.

10. DENIAL FREE BILLING

Any and all services billed to the Facility by the Provider which have been retroactively denied or rejected by governmental agencies or third-party payers will be deducted from the gross amount of the billings of the Provider at such time as all appeals have been exhausted. The Facility will list any deductions from the Provider's billings by patient name and dates of service denied when paying Provider's invoice. Any such denial or rejection which shall be caused by the failure of the Facility or its agents or employees to act in an appropriate manner will be the responsibility of the Facility and not offset against Provider. If the denial or rejection involves an individual claim, Provider's liability to the Facility will be calculated on the basis of specific services denied or rejected.

Facility agrees to promptly notify Provider of any denial received with respect to Provider's services, and provides further, that Provider will be provided a copy of any written denial applicable to Provider's services under this agreement within twenty-one (21) days of the denial's receipt by Facility. Facility agrees that with regard to any denial or rejection, Provider shall have the right to request that Facility appeal said denial or rejection. Provider agrees to provide Facility or its representative with any additional information appropriate to said appeal in a timely manner. Any such amounts previously recovered by the Facility through any appeal or paid under waiver of liability shall be paid to Provider within thirty (30) days of Facility's receipt of said recovered amounts if such amount has for any reason previously been deducted from payment to the Provider.

11. MISCELLANEOUS

Each party to this Agreement acknowledges that no representations, inducement, promises, or agreements, orally or otherwise, have been made by any party, or anyone acting on behalf of any party, which are not embodied herein, and that no other agreement, statement, or promise not contained in this Agreement shall be valid or binding.

Any modification of this Agreement will be effective only if it is in writing and signed by all parties to this Agreement.

IN WITNESS WHEREOF, we the undersigned, duly authorized representatives of the parties to this Agreement herein above expressed, have entered into this Agreement without reservation and have read the terms herein.

Accepted this _____ day of _____, 1998

BY _____
   Facility Representative

BY _____
   Provider Representative

CHAPTER 7

Program Integrity: Documentation and the Written Plan of Care

INTRODUCTION

Documentation is an important aspect of the speech-language pathologist's responsibilities. Documentation is, above all else, written communication. All other verbal or nonverbal communications, when not documented, simply appear never to have occurred. Education, patient and family responses to treatment, and the myriad details of care take on a new importance in the medical record for home care.

This chapter presents guidelines that can assist the speech-language pathologist to document succinctly the treatment given to patients in the home and minimize the time required for that documentation. In addition, basic coverage guidelines are reviewed and documentation for reimbursement is discussed. The initial section of this chapter discusses the medical record, formats, common types of documentation, and actual creation of effective documentation.

THE PRINCIPLES OF DOCUMENTATION: AN OVERVIEW

The practice of speech-language pathology is described in the medical record of any speech-language pathology patient. Speech-language pathology entries that appear in the record reflect the standard of care given by the clinician as well as the particular care given to the specific patient. Other health care team members often make care decisions on the basis of the speech-language pathology notes, especially when they deal with a patient's swallowing problem. Today, many third parties make legal and quality judgments, as well as administrative and reimbursement decisions, and perform other actions peripheral to the actual care of the patient on the basis of that patient's medical record.

Marrelli (1994) states that the typical patient record may be reviewed by a minimum of 10 people during the patient's initial admission into a facility. These individuals may include the physician, three or four nurses, a utilization review specialist, a home health aide, a dietitian, a physical therapist, an occupational therapist, and others. With so many persons depending on the patient's medical record as a reliable source of information on the patient, the importance of documentation contained in the record becomes even more critical.

Documentation is defined as "the supplying of documentary evidence" and "the collecting, abstracting, and coding of printed or written information for future reference" (*Webster's*, 1988, p. 403). This simple definition fits all the varied roles that documentation, or the process of documenting and demonstrating the delivery of care, assumes in health care today. The speech-language pathologist's documentation in the patient's medical record is recognized as a significant contribution that documents the standard of care provided to a patient. As the practice of speech-language pathology has become more complex and more geared toward medical problems in health care, so too have the factors that influence the roles of documentation. These factors include requirements of regulatory agencies, health insurance companies, accreditation organizations, consumers of health care, and legal entities. The speech-language pathologist must try to satisfy these various requirements all at once, often with little time to accomplish this very important task. The speech-language pathologist writing a clinical record entry may need to simultaneously meet the standards of the Joint Commission on Accreditation of Healthcare Organizations, various health insurers, state and federal laws and regulations, and other professional organizations. Fortunately, most home health agencies have integrated many of these requirements, when possible, into agency policy and procedures manuals.

The clinical medical record written today is also the speech-language pathologist's best defense against any litigation in which malpractice or negligence is alleged.

THE INCREASED EMPHASIS ON DOCUMENTATION

The increased specialization of health care providers and the complexity of patient problems and associated technology have contributed to the increase in the amount and the types of services provided to patients. This increased complexity necessitates clear communication among health care team members. The patient's medical record is the only source of written communication, and sometimes the only source of communication, for team members. It is the only document that chronicles a patient's stay from admission through discharge. Team members not only contribute their individual assessments of interventions and outcomes but actually base their subsequent actions on the record of events provided by other team members. All notations must be recorded as soon as possible after the patient's condition changes, an intervention is provided, or a response to treatment is observed. Effective documentation methods demonstrate team work, integrate forms among all disciplines, and allow data to be easily recorded and collated.

Several factors have created an environment in which the speech-language pathologist has increased responsibilities in regard to documentation. The medical record becomes the only written account of these responsibilities and treatment interventions. According to Marrelli (1994), five major factors contribute to the increased emphasis on documentation.

1. *The current economics of the health care system and managed care.* In response to spiraling health care costs, third-party payers have increased their scrutiny and control of agency resources. Payers award health care contracts to those agencies that can control costs, by limiting the patient's length of stay (LOS) and resource utilization, while still providing quality care. In general, decreased LOSs increase patients' speech-language pathology care needs during the shortened time period. The phrase often heard to describe this phenomenon is "quicker and sicker." Third-party payers use the medical record as the basis for payment or denial decisions.

2. *The emphasis on quality or performance improvement in health care.* As quality assurance programs in home health care have evolved, patient outcomes have been recognized as valid indicators of quality care. Clinical documentation demonstrates not only the speech-language pathology services and treatments delivered but the movement toward achieving patient goals and positive outcomes. In addition, the current interdisciplinary focus of quality improvement efforts emphasizes the entire health care team's working to achieve patient-centered care, as well as outcomes. The clinical documentation is the written evidence of this collaboration in the format of team communications, meetings, conferences, and other activities as designated by each home health care agency.

3. *The emphasis on standardization of care and policies and procedures.* All patients are entitled to a certain level or standard of care. As patients and managed care organizations have become more proactive consumers in their purchase of health care services, satisfaction with the care provided becomes a key to a home health agency's reputation and ultimate survival and cost containment. This satisfaction is commonly measured in such factors as patient satisfaction, positive clinical outcomes, and low costs. Speech-language pathologists, because they tend to see patients more frequently than other disciplines do, and usually for longer periods of time, are pivotal to facilitating these success factors. It is also known that satisfied patients are less likely to sue an agency. The role of the speech-language pathologist as patient advocate, listener, and teacher has become widely accepted in recent years.

4. *The increased recognition and empowerment of speech-language pathologists.* Although there are more speech-language pathologists in the work force than ever before, there continues to be a need for qualified speech-language pathologists who are oriented to health care practice and the treatment of medical conditions. The speech-language pathologist's note can become the factor by which documented quality (or negligence) becomes demonstrated quality (or negligence).

5. *The emphasis on effectiveness and efficiency in health care.* As home health care agencies continue to streamline and redesign their operations, the administrative tasks done historically by nurses are being reconsidered. A major focus now is multiskilling of all personnel who make home visits. Repetition or duplication of documentation has been an area of appropriate concern for both the speech-language pathologists and the administrative management of the home health care agencies. Quality, not quantity, is now emphasized with regard to documentation.

DOCUMENTATION GUIDELINES

Speech-language pathology documentation for home health care represents the quality of care provided. Unfortunately, if care is not documented, the assumption can be made that it did not happen. Through complete documentation, the speech-language pathologist can claim credit for meeting responsibilities inherent in the profession. Documentation is a vital adjunct to providing patient care. It is the sole written record of the patient's treatment stay and, as such, represents the care provided. Speech-language pathologists can record clinical care well through thorough, effective, and complete documentation (see Exhibit 7–1). The following tips can be used to improve documentation:

- Write legibly or print neatly. The record must be readable.
- Use permanent ink. (The appropriate ink color may depend on the particular home health care agency.)
- For every entry, identify the time and date, sign the entry with a full signature, and list clinical title.
- Describe the care provided and the patient's response to the care.
- Write objectively in describing any findings.
- Write entries in consecutive and chronological order with no skipped lines or gaps. (This is now a legal requirement in documentation.)
- Write entries as soon after the visit as possible.
- Be factual and specific.
- Use patient, family, and caregiver quotes.
- Use the patient's name (e.g., Mr. Smith).

Exhibit 7–1 Guidelines for Effective Documentation

- Recognize that the speech-language pathologist initiates the process of claims payment (or denial) at the first home care visit.
- Analyze your documentation. Ask yourself if the record of the initial evaluation/visit reflects why the patient is homebound (if the payer has that criterion) and how or why the skills of the speech-language pathologist are needed. Many home health agencies have a peer review process that significantly helps clinicians create and objectively review their own documentation.
- Emphasize the following: (1) why the care was initiated, (2) what the skilled speech-language pathology interventions are, (3) where the patient's plan is going (patient-centered goals), and (4) what the plans are for discharge (rehabilitation potential and outcome).
- Document as soon as possible. Patients understand that there is paperwork associated with health care. Allow a few minutes at the end of each visit for this important task. This is of particular importance when you are working with need missions because of all the associated forms that the patient must sign and the need for correct information to complete the initial and daily visit notes. It can be difficult, and often unsafe, to rely on memory or notes at the end of a long day after seeing many patients.
- Remember that the plan of care (POC) is the most important part of the documentation. All other information flows from the identified skilled needs ordered on the patient POC. The POC or plan of treatment should be either delivered or faxed to the nurse in charge of the case by the next day for inclusion in the HCFA Form 485.
- Make sure that patients meet the home health agency and insurance program admissions criteria. Be able to clearly identify the skilled speech-language pathology services needed and those services that are covered under each particular reimbursement program.
- Focus on the patient's problems in your documentation. Patient problems are why home care is being provided, and the payers must see evidence of such to justify reimbursement.
- Demonstrate through documentation that the care provided is patient centered. For example, ensure that patient goals are quantifiable and that outcomes are realistic, functional, and specific to the patient's unique problems or needs.
- Remember that others who read the patient's clinical record may not have the depth of information and knowledge that you have from actually being there and seeing the patient in his or her home setting. Because of this, documentation information should be objective and should paint a clear picture of the patient and his or her problems and needs and of how the care is directed toward goal achievement and toward discharge and functional outcomes within the home.
- Write succinctly. Effective documentation does not have to be lengthy or wordy. A word of caution: Speech-language pathologists may tend to be verbose. Suc-

continues

Exhibit 7–1 continued

cinct documentation can still convey a lot of information. The documentation, however, should convey to any reader the status of the patient, the adherence to the ordered POC, and consistent movement toward predetermined, patient-centered, functional goals and outcomes.

•. Check that the information in the clinical record flows well and that objective evidence illustrates what is happening with that patient. Information should include the problems and the skilled services that are needed, again based on the full picture presented in the documentation.

• Remember that documentation needs to be legible, neat, and organized consistently. It should include decisions made and explanations. For example, changes in objectives should be explained.

• Document completely to tell the story of the patient's progress (or lack of progress) and the treatment or interventions implemented on the basis of the initial assessment and the patient's POC.

• Document telephone calls and other communications with physicians, community agencies, other team members, and nursing.

• Document what occurred with the patient; what actions were ordered, modified, and implemented; and what the patient's response was to these interventions.

• Demonstrate the speech-language pathology process in a succinct, organized manner in the medical record. Look for the speech-language pathology diagnoses, the assessment, evidence of care planning, implementation of ordered speech-language pathology treatment interventions and actions, movement toward patient-centered functional outcome goals, assessment of the patient's response, and continued evaluation.

• Explain the reasons for any lack of expected progress. If a person is too ill for speech-language pathology services or refuses the service, document your communication with the physician about the problem. Has an order been made to place the service on hold or to discharge the patient from that service?

• Document patient/family/caregiver teaching and their responses to teaching or demonstration of behavior and learning. Document the patient's response to treatment and speech-language pathology interventions.

• Document modifications to the treatment or interventions based on the patient's response, where appropriate.

• Document interdisciplinary team conferences and discussions.

• Demonstrate continuity of care planning goals and consistent movement toward goal achievement by all members of the health care team.

Generally, the medical record should tell the story of the patient's care, needs, and progress and why he or she was receiving speech-language pathology home health care services. It should reflect the level of care expected by today's health care consumers and their families and should demonstrate compliance with regulatory, licensure, and quality standards.

- Document patient complaints or needs and their resolution. Make reference to any consultants used, referrals to nursing, or nursing communication.
- Be complete, accurate, and thorough.
- Write out words. (Avoid potentially confusing abbreviations.)
- Document only care that you have provided.
- Promptly document a change in the patient's condition and the actions taken based on that change. Be sure to record all changes also in the patient care plan and communicate with the nurse and physician if necessary.
- Write the patient's, family's, or caregiver's response to teaching or home educational programs.
- Correct entries properly: (1) Draw a single line through the erroneous entry; (2) briefly describe the error (e.g., wrong day, wrong chart); and (3) add signature, date, and time.
- Do not rely on memory.
- Do not white out or erase entries.
- Do not cross out words beyond recognition.
- Do not make assumptions, draw conclusions, or blame others.
- Do not leave blank spaces on narrative notes between entries and the signature.
- Do not leave gaps in documentation.
- Do not use abbreviations, except where they are clear and appear on the agency's list of acceptable abbreviations.

Exhibit 7–2 provides a checklist for reviewing documentation.

DOCUMENTING THE PLAN OF CARE

Standards of Care

There are many professional standards of care and areas of practice for speech-language pathology. The following guidelines for standards of care have proven to be acceptable by the health care profession.

Standard 1: Assessment

Standard. The speech-language pathologist collects patient health data.

Measurement Criteria.
- The priority of data collection is determined by the patient's immediate condition or needs.
- Pertinent data are collected using appropriate assessment techniques and diagnostic tests.

Exhibit 7–2 Checklist for Documentation

_____ Does the documentation tell the story of the patient's progress or lack of progress and the treatment implemented on the basis of the speech-language pathology evaluation?

_____ Are telephone calls and other communications with physicians or other team members documented?

_____ Does the documentation explain what happened: what actions were taken, ordered, and carried out, and the patient's response to care?

_____ Are acceptable standards of speech-language pathology practice demonstrated? Look for the speech-language pathology diagnoses, the written assessment, and the evidence of care planning, implementation of the interventions, and assessment of the patient's response and further evaluation.

_____ Is there documentation of goal achievement and/or progress toward goals and outcomes?

_____ Are the goals realistic, measurable, and clear to other readers?

_____ If progress has not occurred as planned, are the reasons for this clearly stated?

_____ Is the patient's response to patient care, treatment, or actions described? For example, when home exercises or motor strengthening has occurred, is the response to these home exercises documented?

_____ Is there documentation that treatments were modified on the basis of the patient's response, where appropriate?

_____ Is there written communication among multidisciplinary team members regarding patient goals and outcomes?

_____ Does the documentation show continuity of care and further coordination based on changing needs of the patient?

_____ Does the medical record represent current professional speech-language pathology standards of practice?

_____ Is the medical record neat and legible?

_____ Generally, does the documentation tell the story of the patient's treatment by the speech-language pathologist?

_____ Does the documentation make sense, with no unexplained gaps?

_____ Does the documentation show that actions of team members have been directed toward the same goals?

_____ Does the documentation show that actions by the speech-language pathologist contribute to the patient's receiving care that will assist in meeting the stated goals and outcomes?

_____ Does the documentation show that speech-language pathology actions are focused on identifying discharge goals or outcomes, for example, how the family or significant others are involved in care, whether they have input into the plan, and whether they are being taught about the individual care?

_____ Does the documentation reflect speech-language pathology treatment at the level expected by today's consumer?

- Data collection involves the patient, significant others, and other health care providers, when appropriate.
- The data collection is systematic and ongoing.
- Relevant data are documented in a retrievable form and communicated to all parties who have influence in the overall care of the patient.

Standard 2: Diagnosis

Standard. The speech-language pathologist analyzes the diagnostic test data in determining diagnoses.

Measurement Criteria.
- Diagnoses are derived from the diagnostic tests and assessment data.
- Diagnoses are validated with the patient, significant others, and other health care providers when possible.
- Diagnoses are documented in a manner that facilitates the determination of expected outcomes and the patient POC.

Standard 3: Outcome Identification

Standard. The speech-language pathologist identifies specific outcomes individualized to the patient.

Measurement Criteria.
- Outcomes are derived from the diagnoses.
- Outcomes are documented as measurable goals.
- Outcomes are mutually formulated with the patient, other health care providers and team members, and family and/or caregivers when possible.
- Outcomes are realistic in relation to the patient's present and potential capabilities.
- Outcomes are obtainable in relation to resources available to the patient and to family and/or caregiver abilities.
- Outcomes include a time estimate for attainment.
- Outcomes provide direction for continuity of care and discharge planning.

Standard 4: Planning

Standard. The speech-language pathologist develops a POC that prescribes treatment to attain the expected outcomes.

Measurement Criteria.
- The POC is individualized to the patient's condition or needs.
- The plan is developed with the patient, family, and/or caregiver and other health care team members when appropriate.
- The POC reflects current speech-language pathology practice.

- The plan is documented.
- The plan provides for continuity of care and discharge planning.

Standard 5: Treatment

Standard. The speech-language pathologist implements the treatment or treatments identified in the POC.

Measurement Criteria.
- Interventions are consistent with the established POC.
- Interventions are implemented in a safe and appropriate manner.
- Interventions are documented.
- Interventions are geared toward functional communication and the patient's ability to function independently in his or her environment.

Standard 6: Evaluation

Standard. The speech-language pathologist evaluates the patient's progress toward attainment of outcomes.

Measurement Criteria.
- Evaluation is systematic, consistent, and ongoing.
- The patient's responses to treatment are documented well.
- The effectiveness of treatment is evaluated in relation to outcomes and the overall patient care plan.
- Assessment is an ongoing process, and the clinician uses ongoing assessment data to revise outcomes, POCs, and treatment modalities as needed.
- Revisions to outcomes in the POC are documented.
- The patient's significant others and/or family and health care providers are involved in the evaluation process when appropriate.

Frequency and Length-of-Stay Considerations

The frequency of visits and the length of service are usually based on the speech-language pathologist's assessment or ongoing evaluation of the patient's clinical status, as well as on the unique speech-language pathology/communication deficits and unique family systems needs. The clinician must remember that all visits require orders by the physician, and the speech-language pathologist must maintain compliance with Medicare Conditions of Participation, state licensure, surveyor directives, and other regulations or laws.

Experienced home health speech-language pathologists know that they are in an important position to identify the patient's specific service and visit frequency needs. The objective findings, as found through the speech-language pathology assessment, are the basis for recommendations made by the speech-language pathologist and communicated to the physician. Some patients may be seen infrequently by their physician after discharge and may lack adequate transportation to the physician's office. Physicians sometimes do not make needed home health visits to homebound patients. Decisions about visit frequency are therefore dependent on speech-language pathologist judgment skills. The *Health Insurance Manual-11* (HIM-11) states the following about frequency in the text addressing the completion of element 21 on the Health Care Financing Administration (HCFA) Form 485: "Frequency denotes the number of visits per discipline to be rendered, stated in days, weeks, or months. Duration identifies the length of time the services are to be rendered and may be expressed in days, weeks, or months" (HCFA, 1989). In home care, *duration* usually refers to the LOS for which the patient is projected to need home care services in order to safely and effectively meet the patient's unique medical and other needs. Realistically and operationally, other factors—besides medical or speech-language pathology practice standards—are important to scheduling and frequency decisions, such as staffing trends, standards of practice, geographic location of the patient, family and referral support systems, and the availability of qualified staff for patients with particular conditions or problems. When conflict occurs between patient needs and the speech-language pathologist's ability to meet those needs, other courses of action should be implemented. Various factors are considered in the process of determining frequency and duration of care.

A general rule of thumb for frequency, which is required by most home health care agencies, is that patients are not scheduled for more than three visits weekly. The rationale from the HCFA is that when a patient needs rehabilitative care more than three times a week, the patient should probably be referred to an inpatient facility for more intensive therapy. Although daily therapy is a very accepted standard of practice for home health nursing practice and home health aide practice, it is very uncommon for speech-language pathology care. There are instances, on occasion, in which five-day-a-week therapy is warranted and through appropriate documentation can be justified. For example, a patient who is at risk for aspiration pneumonia may be seen for a very limited time on a daily basis. Typically, the LOS is no more than five times weekly for two weeks. Another "quirk" in the system is that Medicare clearly frowns on speech-language pathology or any type of rehabilitative care being given on consecutive days. It appears that intermediaries feel that patients need time to recover from a therapeutic regimen, and they therefore require that a day be skipped between treatments. The only exception to this rule is during holidays, patient vacations, or patient illness, when visits need to be made up.

Practice guidelines, outcome measures, and standards of care are important because of the increased emphasis on cost-effective, high-quality care. These practice parameters will help the home health speech-language pathologist to determine patient frequency and length of time in service. Speech-language pathologists working in home health care must be flexible and able to explain objective reasons for frequency, LOS, and discharge decisions. These decisions and their underlying rationale need to be communicated clearly to the home health agency and to third-party payer representatives who are responsible for tracking, approving, or denying visits. As payers try to decrease the number of patient visits, the speech-language pathologist must be able to articulate the clinical needs of the patient and be a patient advocate for high-quality home care. Advocacy is more important now as the technology explosion continues and speech-language pathologists care for patients with more difficult conditions in the home, such as patients receiving ventilator care and patients with swallowing and feeding deficits. Clinicians who can explain patient needs on the basis of objective information and patient findings to the numerous reimbursement gatekeepers will continue to be successful in the home health care arena. The increasing complexity of patients sent home with limited resources and coverage demands those skills for safe and effective patient care.

Documenting the Written Plan of Treatment

A clear understanding of the guidelines for documentation of speech-language pathology services provided in the home health setting will assist the speech-language pathologist to provide reimbursable, quality home care to individuals. Documentation is the key, the reward is reimbursement, and the result is care provided to patients in need of the service. Appendix 7–A contains excerpts from the Interpretive Guidelines for Speech-Language Pathology developed by the HCFA, Region IV. Appendix 7–B provides a description of speech-language pathology services, and Appendix 7–C shows an example of a comprehensive functional outcome assessment.

CONCLUSION

Home care is the fastest-growing segment of health care. Speech-language pathologists are acutely aware of the changes and advances in technology that have influenced the kinds of patients now seen in the home setting. The home care speech-language pathologists of the present and future must be service oriented, flexible, and clinically strong. Payers and insurers must continue to address spiraling health care costs. The historic and customary way to approach these rising costs has been to decrease authorized vists/services or to add additional review levels. It is the professional home care speech-language pathologist who can validate the need for skilled speech-language pathology care and back it up by effective documentation.

REFERENCES

Health Care Financing Administration. (1989). *Medicare home health agency manual* (Publication No. HIM-11). Baltimore: Author.

Marrelli, T.M. (1994). *Handbook of home health standards and documentation guidelines for reimbursement* (2nd ed.). St. Louis, MO: Mosby.

Webster's New World Dictionary (3rd ed.). (1988). New York: Simon & Schuster.

SUGGESTED READING

American Nurses' Association. (1992). *Standards of home health nursing practice.* Washington, DC: Author.

American Occupational Therapy Association. (1995). *Guidelines for occupational therapy practice in home health.* Bethesda, MD: Author.

Benner, P., & Tanner, C. (1987). Clinical judgement: How expert nurses use intuition. *American Journal of Nursing.*

Collopy, B., Dubler, N., & Zuckerman, C. (1990). The ethics of home care: Autonomy and accommodation. *The Hastings Center Report, 20*(2, Suppl.), 3.

Gottrred, C.H. (1987). *Intermediary interpretative review guidelines for speech-language pathology and audiology services.* Washington, DC: Health Care Financing Administration, Region V, Division of Health, Standards and Quality.

Health Care Financing Administration. (1990). *Medicare intermediary manual,* Part 3, *Claims process* (DHHS Transmittal No. 1487, Section 3906.4). Washington, DC: U.S. Government Printing Office.

Humphrey, C.J. (1988). The home as a setting for care: Clarifying the boundaries of practice. *Nursing Clinics of North America, 22*(2), 305–314.

Interpretive Guidelines for Speech-Language Pathology

PHYSICIAN OR SPEECH-LANGUAGE PATHOLOGIST WRITTEN PLAN OF TREATMENT

As of January 1, 1981, the addition of the following paragraph was made to 3148.3. It should be assumed this applies to all provider settings.

Effective January 1, 1981, for outpatient speech pathology services and effective July 18, 1984, for outpatient physical therapy services, such services also may be furnished under a written plan of treatment established by the speech pathologist providing such speech pathology services or by the qualified physical therapist providing such physical therapy services; however, the plan must be periodically reviewed by the physician. The speech pathologist's or physical therapist's plan must be established (that is, reduced to writing by that pathologist or physical therapist or by the provider itself when it makes a written record of the pathologist's or physical therapist's oral orders) before treatment is begun. Such plans should be promptly signed by the pathologist or physical therapist providing such services and incorporated into the provider's permanent record for the patient. Plan of treatment for outpatient speech language pathology or outpatient physical therapy services established by the speech pathologist or physical therapist providing such services must also relate the type, amount, frequency, and duration of the speech pathology or physical therapy services that are to be furnished the patient and indicate the diagnosis and anticipated goals.

Source: Adapted from Region 5 Guidelines, Health Care Financing Administration.

Any changes to a plan established by the speech pathologist or physical therapist must be made in writing and signed by that pathologist or physical therapist or by the attending physician. Changes to such plans may be made pursuant to the oral orders given by the attending physician, as stated above, or by the pathologist to another qualified physical therapist or a registered professional nurse on the staff of the provider. Such changes must be immediately recorded in the patient's records and signed by the individual receiving the orders. While the physician may change a plan of treatment established by the speech pathologist or qualified physical therapist providing such services, the speech pathologist may not alter a plan of treatment established by a physician.

REASONABLE AND NECESSARY: LEVEL OF COMPLEXITY

Decisions on level of complexity should be based on what the speech-language pathologist does, not necessarily what it appears that the patient is asked to do. For example, the patient may be asked to repeat a word and the pathologist analyzes the response and gives the patient feedback in order that the patient modifies the response. The speech-language pathologist may ask staff or family to repeat the activity with the patient as a reinforcement; however, it is the speech-language pathologist's sophisticated analysis that makes the activity skilled. Medicare will not pay for repetitive artic exercises.

QUALIFIED SPEECH-LANGUAGE PATHOLOGIST

Speech pathologist or audiologist (qualified consultant). A person who is licensed, if applicable, by the State in which practicing, and (1) Is eligible for a certificate of clinical competence in the appropriate area (speech language pathology or audiology) granted by the American Speech and Hearing Association under its requirements in effect on the publication of this provision; or (2) Meets the educational requirements for certification, and is in the process of accumulating the supervised experience required for certification.

Speech-language pathologists or audiologists should indicate their certification status by using CCC-Sp, CCC-A, CFY:

CCC-Sp   Certificate of Clinical Competence—Speech-Language Pathology
CCC-A   Certificate of Clinical Competence—Audiology
CFY   Clinical Fellowship Year

SIGNIFICANT PROGRESS

Significant progress means that the patient will "improve significantly in a reasonable (and generally predictable) period of time." The reporting of progress is of extreme importance. The speech-language pathologist should provide adequate information of the overall treatment plan and goals. Documentation of progress toward a functional goal should be available. This documentation should contain objective data. *The treatment plan and chosen measures should remain the same over the entire duration of treatment unless a need for change is explained by the speech-language pathologist.*

AMOUNT, FREQUENCY, AND DURATION OF SERVICES

Estimates of session numbers and months per diagnosis are available; however, these are not limits but guidelines of averages and ranges reported by speech-language pathologists. The reviewer *must not use these as limits* to length of reimbursement. There must be functional goals related back to the patient's medical condition.

PROVIDER INFORMATION

(All information must be typed or printed and must be readable even if Xeroxed.) In addition to provider/beneficiary identification information, most intermediaries now require:

- Medical diagnosis
- Communicative disorder diagnosis
- Date of onset
- Medical history
- Length of treatment time
- Number of times treatment rendered
- Narrative progress
- Number of treatments to date
- Date patient began at present facility

The following are either clarifications of the above categories or additional categories that may be requested in order to facilitate claims review.

1. *Date of onset.* This is to reflect date of trauma, CVA, surgery, etc. In lieu of one of these, as in the case of progressive disease (Multiple Sclerosis, Amyotrophic Lateral Sclerosis, Parkinsonism), the date of onset would be the date of the original diagnosis by physician. Indicate date speech problem began.

2. *Date of original speech language evaluation.* This will reflect the date (or approximate date) of the first speech language evaluation completed for the *present* medical disorder regardless of setting. Therefore, the provider would report the date of an evaluation that may have been completed at a previous provider setting. There are instances that the provider may not have access to this date. For example, if a patient has had two strokes, this date would reflect the date of the speech language evaluation that took place after the second stroke regardless if an evaluation had been done after the first stroke.

NOTE: This may be significantly separate from the date of onset in the case of progressive neurologic disease where the speech language disorder may not appear for months or years after disease onset.

3. *Date of initial treatment.* This would reflect the date of the original treatment. This might be separate from the original evaluation for many reasons, i.e.,
   a. Original evaluation did not indicate that treatment would be beneficial at the time.
   b. Patient left the original meeting.
   c. Patient refused treatment until present.

4. *Length of prior treatment to the present provider setting, if possible.* Indication of amount of the treatment in previous provider setting, if possible, in history.

5. *Functional goals and status.* A functional goal should be written by the speech language pathologist that reflects the level of communicative independence the patient is *expected* to achieve outside of the therapeutic environment. Therefore, this goal should:
   a. Reflect the final level the patient is expected to achieve
   b. Be the end result of the treatment plan
   c. Be a realistic goal
   d. Reflect *functional* change in the patient's ability to communicate outside the therapy environment .
   e. Have a positive effect on the quality of patient's everyday life

It is assumed that certain factors may change, thus increasing or decreasing the final level of achievement. However, if this occurs, the speech language pathologist should explain the factors that led to the change of functional goal. *The following are examples of functional communication goals which the patient may progress through to achieve optimum communication independence.* The term "communication" as used below refers to both expressive and receptive skills and includes both verbal and nonverbal modalities.
   a. Ability to communicate basic physical needs and emotional status as well as comprehension of simple questions requiring a yes/no response
   b. Ability to communicate basic *activities of daily living needs*
   c. Ability to engage in social communicative interaction with immediate family and/or those who are very familiar with the patient

    d. Ability to carry out communicative interactions in the community

    e. Ability to carry out avocation or vocational communication needs

The provider *must* report all four of the following:

    a. Initial status at this provider setting

    b. Present status for this reporting period

    c. Demonstrated progress

    d. Potential for rehabilitation

Note that a functional goal may reflect small but meaningful change which enables the patient to function more *independently* in a reasonable amount of time. For instance, for some patients, it may be reflected in the ability to give a consistent functional "yes" and "no" response; for others, it may be the use of gestures to convey needs. Some may be able to use an alternate mode of communication such as a picture communication book, alphabet board or electronic communication device; others may be able to use such alternate communication systems plus a few spoken words. Some may be able to receptively and expressively use a basic spoken vocabulary and/or short phrases; others may regain the ability of conversational language skills and still others may refine their conversational language skills and still others may refine their conversational speech skills to a level acceptable in a normal active environment. *The critical factor is that the patient is able to communicate in a more significant and functional manner as a result of speech pathology treatment than prior to such treatment.*

    6. *Progress.* It is essential that the provider includes not only a short narrative progress report but gives some type of *objective information in a clear and concise manner at least every 30 days.* This should be done in such a manner that the reviewer has access to the entire plan of treatment, along with any changes in the goals or treatment plan. *The reviewer should have access to an overall treatment plan with final goals and enough objective information to determine progress toward these goals.*

The following components would be required:

    a. *Functional goals:* A goal written by the speech language pathologist reflecting the pathologist's judgment as to the patient's restorative potential. It will be written in terms of how the patient will function outside of the therapeutic environment.

    b. *Speech/language goals:* Goals written to subserve the functional goal. When the patient achieves these goals, the functional goal would be the result.

NOTE: *It is very important for the reviewer to be given a clear understanding of the purpose and the final goal of treatment.*

If the speech-language pathologist reports that the patient can produce an /m/ 25% of the time, then 40%, then 60%, then 90%, the reviewer is led to believe the patient is making progress. However, the clinician must also interpret these percentages into how this treatment has made the patient independent in communication. Percentages will no longer stand alone. However, if the reviewer is given the ultimate goal and the intervening speech language goals, then one can see the progress toward the final goal as well as the interrelationship between the final goal and the goals subservient to that final goal. For example, the speech-language pathologist might state that the final goal is "the ability to converse in a limited environment." One underlying speech language goal might be "to reduce the apraxia sufficiently in order that the patient can initiate short intelligible phrases with a minimum of apraxic errors." The short-term goals or a step-by-step treatment plan would demonstrate that working on the patient's ability to initiate certain easier phonemes would come before working on other phonemes which the patient found more difficult. (This might be due to an inability to neurologically program speech musculature.)

Therefore, the speech-language pathologist has a linguistically and neurologically sound basis for working on one phoneme production before initiating another.

The pathologist also might choose to work on a group of phonemes having a feature in common before working on another group, for example, working on all bilabials, since the patient can easily see the movement, then moving to sounds that are produced more intraorally.

The reviewer might not be knowledgeable of the bases of speech language pathology procedures but if given an overall plan of treatment, would be able to judge whether or not progress is being made toward the completion of the plan.

    c. *Demonstration of Progress*: The speech language pathologist may choose how to demonstrate progress. *However, the method chosen as well as the measures used must remain the same over the duration of treatment. The concept of reporting progress consistently is extremely important.* If the reviewer is given an overview of the *purpose* and *goal* of treatment and can compare the patient's status in the present reporting period with that of the previous reporting period, the reviewer will be able to make a correct reimbursement decision. For example, if the speech language pathologist reports a subtest score one month, then a score of a different subtest the next month without demonstrating either the goals of the subtests or their interrelation, the reviewer will not be able to judge the progress, if any, that these differences represent. These claims may either be denied or returned to the provider for additional information.

    7. *Signature.* Signature of a speech language pathologist or audiologist should be followed by:

CCC-SP   Certified speech-language pathologist

CCC-A   Certified audiologist
CFY-Sp   Clinical Fellowship Year—Speech-Language Pathology
CFY-A   Clinical Fellowship Year—Audiology
(CFY can perform reimbursable coverage under proper supervision by a certified speech language pathologist or audiologist.)

REPORTING ON NEW EPISODE OR CONDITION

Occasionally, a patient who is presently receiving or has previously received speech language services experiences a new illness or new episode of an illness. The provider must document the significance of any change to the communication capabilities of the patient. This may be demonstrated by pre and post episode objective documentation and/or scores, by nursing notes, or by physician reports. If the patient is presently receiving treatment, treatment would not be lengthened unless it was to accommodate an interruption in service or the reviewer has access to documentation verifying a change in communication status. If the patient has completed treatment for the original communication deficit, a significant change in the communication status must be documented to warrant initiation of a new treatment plan.

Skilled versus Unskilled Procedures

Skilled Procedures	Unskilled Procedures
Diagnostic and evaluation services to ascertain the type, causal factor(s) and severity of speech and language disorders. Re-evaluation if the patient exhibits a change in functional speech or motivation, clearing of confusion, or remission of some other medical condition which previously contraindicated speech pathology.	Non-diagnostic/non-therapeutic routine, repetitive and reinforced procedures (e.g., the practicing of word drills without sophisticated and skilled feedback).
Evaluation and diagnosis of the speech and/or language disorder, or any related disorder.	Procedures which may be repetitive and/or reinforcing of *previously* learned material which staff or family may be instructed to repeat.
Design of a treatment program relevant to the patient's disorder(s). Continued assessment of patient's progress during the implementation of such treatment program, including: documentation and professional analysis of patient's status at regular intervals.	Procedures which may be reviewed with patient by any non-professional (i.e., family member, restorative nursing aide, etc.).
Establishing a hierarchy of tasks and a hierarchy of cueing that works patient toward communication goals.	Tallying of transfer practice outside treatment.
Establishing compensatory skills (e.g., air-injection techniques, word-finding strategies).	Making right/wrong decisions (probably not quality of response judgments).
Making judgments related to actual progress within goals.	Providing practice for use of augmentative or alternative communication systems.
Selecting and establishing augmentative/alternative communication devices.	(NOTE: It is only after the patient has established a high level of consistency of performance in a task with the speech language pathologist that unskilled techniques can be implemented.)
Establishing transfer strategies for augmentative communication systems.	

Statements Supporting and Not Supporting Continued Care

Statements Supporting Continued Care	Statements NOT (of themselves) Supportive of Continued Care
Typically these statements should have an objective component, which is *compared to previous reporting*, and which demonstrates *progress toward a stated functional goal.*	These statements may be appropriate in a progress report; however, narrative should also contain reference to objective scoring, comparison of previous scores, or treatment plan with present status compared to previous status. This information could be imbedded in narrative or attached; however, the reviewer should have access to this information and *stated functional goal.*
Good examples: "Mr. Smith achieved 76 on the Word Subtest of the Johnson Test of Aphasia compared with last month's score of 50 on the same Subtest."	*Bad examples:* "Mrs. Jones very concerned about going home. She has begun smoking again which is causing family problems as well as physical problems."
"Mr. Jones achieved a combined score of 352 on the A, B, C, D, and E subtests this month compared with an overall score of 250 for these *SAME* subtests last month."	"Speech somewhat slurred today." "Mr. Smith more consistent in responses."
"Mrs. Jones achieved the next step in the treatment plan outlined last month (see attached sheet). If she continues at this rate, she should complete treatment within the next 2 months."	"Mr. Jones has shown significant improvement in his ability to make himself understood." "Patient is now able to inject air 80% of the time."
"Mrs. Jones achieved 75% (7.5 out of 10 or 75 out of 100) on word naming task. This compares to last month's score of 50% (50 out of 100)."	"Mrs. Smith achieved 75% accuracy on word naming task." (*No comparison to previous report.*)
(NOTE: % should be based on real number count.)	"Auditory comprehension improved from mildly impaired to moderately impaired." (By itself, does not offer sufficient objective information. Need to compare to previous month.)

LENGTH OF TREATMENT GUIDES

The following reviews some commonly occurring speech language disorders along with reasons justifying varying lengths of treatment for each type of disorder.

These guides are NOT LIMITS to length of treatment but are meant to ease review of claims. Final determination of treatment length should be made by continuation of SIGNIFICANT PROGRESS.

The sessions referred to are the typical 45 to 60 minute session lengths. Typically, patients are seen once a day for 30, 45, or 60 minute sessions. Sometimes patients are seen for shorter periods and several times a day (e.g., three 10-minute sessions, total of 30 minutes). Rarely expected during an evaluation are session lengths longer than 60 minutes. If longer times are noted, the speech language pathologist should justify the time by noting that the patient is exceptionally alert, the number of appropriate activities is great with all activities needing skilled intervention, or special staff/family training is required.

If the patient is an inpatient there also may be further exceptions, since intensive treatment is sometimes required immediately post operatively (e.g., Tracheoesophageal puncture) or postonset of disorder (due to intensive family involvement).

The American Speech-Language-Hearing Association's 1985 Omnibus Survey reported the following as average session's definitions:

Average Length of Time in Minutes	*% of Responses*
15	2.5%
20	11.5%
30	48.5%
45	11.2%
60	11.6%
90	.8%

Source: Reprinted from Region 5 Guidelines, Health Care Financing Administration.

Aural Rehabilitation
(Lip-Reading/Speech Reading)

Typical length of treatment for adult groups—6 to 8 weeks, one session per week

- may continue if significant functional progress continues
- usually not more than 12 sessions

Pre-Testing

1. Basic hearing evaluation:
   (not covered unless information required by physician for determination of further medical procedure)
2. Hearing aid evaluation (HAE)
   (not covered)
3. Speech discrimination in quiet and in noise
   - phoneme level
   - word level
   - sentence level

Pre- and Post-Testing

Speech reading/lip-reading test (may do some of the following):

- Consonant Confusion Test
- Utley Test
- Central Institute for the Deaf (CID)
- The Everyday Speech Sentences
- Testing of combined auditory-visual processing as well as testing lip reading ability only
- Hearing Performance Inventory*
- Denver Scale of Communication Function*
- Denver Scale for Senior Citizens Living in Nursing Homes*
- Hearing Handicap Scale*
- Hearing Handicap Index for the Elderly
- Communication Profile for the Hearing Impaired

*These scales are especially effective in demonstrating functional progress.

Most good candidates for aural rehabilitation treatment are individuals who are alert, non-aphasic, have adequate visual acuity, some residual hearing (aided or unaided), and adequate memory skills. For example, if the patient cannot follow directions, or does not have adequate visual acuity even with glasses to observe lip movements, prognosis for improvement will be inadequate to support reimbursement.

Either Audiologists or Speech-Language Pathologists may provide this service.

Source: Reprinted from Region 5 Guidelines, Health Care Financing Administration.

Dysphasia—Swallowing Disorders

Typical Diagnoses:

Neurologic:

- CVA
- Parkinson
- Multiple Sclerosis

The act of swallowing may be thought of in 4 steps:

1) Preparation Stage:
   - Mastication
   - Bolus Formation
2) Oral Stage: Bolus on dorsum of tongue, tip stabilized on alveolar ridge, peristaltic motion waves bolus through facial pillars
3) Pharyngeal Stage: Bolus is carried by peristaltic wave from facial pillars through cricopharyngeal sphincter, while velum is closed, larynx is elevated, epiglottis eflects, cricopharyngeous relaxes.
4) Esophageal Stage: Continued peristaltic motion carries bolus from cricopharyngeous through gastric sphincter.

Source: Reprinted with permission from Region 5 Guidelines, Health Care Financing Administration.

The first three stages may be especially compliant to treatment intervention thereby increasing the patient's oral intake and quality of life and reducing the need in some cases for surgical intervention.

Often a videofluoroscopic examination of the swallow is performed by the radiologist and the speech language pathologist to determine the amount of aspiration, stage and type of disorder (e.g., vallecular stasis) and possible therapeutic intervention (e.g., aspiration decreases when patient turns head effectively closing one pyriform sinus).

When a videofluoroscopic evaluation is not warranted or not feasible, the speech language pathologist performs a "bedside" swallow evaluation. He or she may then determine whether or not treatment is warranted or that he or she will need a videofluoroscopic evaluation to continue safely. Treatment may be delayed until the evaluation is possible.

Dysphasia treatment often consists of two or three short periods a day. Typically the total treatment time in one day does not exceed sixty minutes. Many patients only require an evaluation with suggestions to the staff or family. Others requiring intervention do not typically exceed two months of treatment.

The following memo clarifies the policy regarding the need for a concomitant speech language disorder. It was sent from Region IX to their Part A Intermediaries.

> It has come to our attention that some intermediaries are making incorrect coverage determinations on claims which involve speech pathology services for the treatment of dysphasia.
>
> Speech pathology services are those services necessary for the diagnosis and treatment of speech and language disorders which result in communication disabilities. The evaluation and treatment of *dysphasia* are covered when performed by a speech pathologist.
>
> . . . Each intermediary should review its procedures for processing these types of claims. Claims should not be denied where the conditions above are met. Claims should also not be approved where there is not a communication disorder.

Head Trauma

Head trauma may cause neurologically based speech language or swallowing disorders. However, the pattern of recovery may differ from etiologies such as CVA. The severity of the communicative disorder may range from extremely mild to extremely severe. In many cases, both the language dominant hemisphere as well as the non-dominant hemisphere is involved. While longer treatment may be warranted for head trauma cases, many are under sixty-five years of age.

Types of Disorders Typically NOT Covered for the Geriatric Patient
1. *Stuttering (except neurogenic stuttering caused by acquired brain damage)*
   Fluency Disorder
   Cluttering
   Disprosody
   Disfluency
2. *Myofunctional Disorders*
   Tongue thrusting
3. *Any Congenital Disorders*—unless there has been no previous treatment, the patient's communicative or swallowing capabilities have deteriorated, or new techniques or instruments are available; however, the reviewer should carefully note the documentation of potential for significant improvement.

List of Reasons It May Be Appropriate To Dismiss a Patient from Or Not Initiate Treatment with a Possibility of Later Reinstatement

Examples:

Reasons To Dismiss	Reasons To Resume
1. Global Aphasia/no progress	Patient's prognosis changes
	Patient becomes more attentive
2. Aphasia that had stabilized	Patient is reported by physician or family to show change in linguistic behavior
3. Any head and neck cancer surgery patient with reaction to radiation or chemotherapy making treatment not viable	Reaction to radiation or chemotherapy is reduced to a degree that therapy will again be beneficial
4. Degenerative central nervous system disorders, i.e., Parkinsonism Multiple Sclerosis Amyotrophic Lateral Sclerosis	Some patients' speech disorder symptoms not significant until long post onset of disease
5. Depression	Response to treatment increased mental state (improved)
6. Transfer or environmental change	New placement has stimulated change in patient's motivation for treatment or in linguistic capabilities themselves
7. Medical problems preclude benefit from treatment intervening illness	Medical problems cleared
8. Intermittent comatose condition	Patient is alert
9. Inability to physically tolerate treatment	Tolerance improves
10. Lack of family support/carry-over	Support system improves
11. No previous insurance coverage	Medicare eligible

Examples of Positive and Negative Prognostic Indicators
for Treatment Candidates

1. Level of alertness: high -- low
2. Severity of deficit: mild -- severe
3. Family involvement: high --- low
4. Patient motivation: high -- low
5. Complicating medical factors: none -------------------------------- many
6. Complicating psychological factors: none -------------------------- many
7. Education level: high --- low
8. Premorbid functional level: high ----------------------------------- low
9. Awareness/acceptance of deficit: good --------------------------- poor
10. Socio-economic: high -- low
11. Chemical dependency
12. Fatigue
13. Heavy medication
14. Extreme chronic lability
15. Dementia
16. Weather/transportation problem

Usually Covered Diagnoses

- Aphasia
- Dysarthria
- Apraxia
- Laryngectomy
- Glossectomy
- Non-dominant Hemisphere Language Impairment (Rt. CVA)

The above diagnoses are usually covered if the patient is eligible and progress continues to be made.

Complicating Factors That May DECREASE Amount of Treatment

- Patient's Lack of Cooperation
- Lack of Transportation
- Medical Complications
- Co-Insurance Expense
- Physician Does Not Refer in Timely Manner
- Bilingual Patient
- Denial of Problem by Patient or Family
- Lack of Motivation
- Decreased Alertness, Lethargy
- Depression

Complicating Factors That May INCREASE Amount of Treatment

- Multiple Disorders
- Fatigue/Decreased Endurance
- Waiting for Other Care Plan Factors (i.e., Augmentative Equipment, Dentures, Hearing Aid)
- Medical Complication
- Cognitive Deficit Due to Traumatic Brain Injury
- Availability of Speech-Language Pathologist

New Procedures in Field

(But not still experimental)
- Tracheo-esophageal Puncture
- Augmentative Communication Systems
- Treatment of Ventilator Dependent Patient

APPENDIX 7–B

Speech-Language
Pathology Services

Medicare Intermediary Manual (Part A), HIM-13, 3101.10A
Description of coverage of services for Speech-Language Pathology is found in
the following provider manuals, as well as 3101.10A.

Provider Manual	Section Number
Medicare Intermediary (Part A), HIM-13	3101.10A
Skilled Nursing Facility, HIM-12	230.3
Hospital, HIM-10	210.11
Home Health Agency, HIM-11	205.3
Medicare Carrier (Part B), HIM-14	2216
Outpatient Physical Therapy, HIM-9	205.6

These description are essentially the same. Any additions are noted in the following.

3101.10A Speech Pathology Services Furnished by the Hospital or by Others under Arrangements with the Hospital and under Its Supervision.

1. *General.* Speech pathology services are those services necessary for the diagnosis and treatment of speech and language disorders which result in communication disabilities. They must relate directly and specifically to a written treatment

Source: Adapted from *Intermediary Interpretive Review Guidelines for Speech Language Pathology and Audiology,* Region 5, Division of Health Standards and Quality, Health Care Financing Administration.

regimen established by the physician after any needed consultation with the qualified speech pathologist.

2. *Reasonable and Necessary.* Speech pathology services must be reasonable
and necessary to the treatment of the individual's illness or injury. To be considered reasonable and necessary, the following conditions must be met:

a. The services must be considered under accepted standards of practice to be
   a specific and effective treatment for the patient's condition.

b. The services must be of such a level of complexity and sophistication, or
   the patient's condition must be such that the required services can be safely
   and effectively performed only by or under the supervision of a qualified
   speech pathologist. (See 42 CFR 405.1202 (u) (1) (2).) When the intermediary determines the services furnished were of a type that could have been
   safely and effectively performed only by qualified speech pathologists or
   under the supervision of a qualified speech pathologist, it should presume
   that such services were properly supervised. However, this assumption is
   rebuttable and, if in the course of processing claims the intermediary finds
   that speech pathology services are not being furnished under proper supervision, the intermediary should deny the claim and bring this matter to the
   attention of the Division of Health Standards and Quality of the HCFA
   Regional Office.

c. There must be an expectation that the patient's condition will improve significantly in a reasonable (and generally predictable) period of time based
   on the assessment by the physician of the patient's restoration potential
   after any needed consultation with the qualified speech pathologist, or the
   services must be necessary to the establishment of a safe and effective
   maintenance program required in connection with a specific disease state;
   and

d. The amount, frequency, and duration of the services must be reasonable
   under accepted standards of practice. (The intermediary should consult
   with local speech pathologists or the State chapter of the American Speech-
   Language-Hearing Association in the development of any utilization
   guidelines.)

Claims for speech pathology services, which are not reasonable and necessary,
should be considered denied under authority of section 1862 (u) (1) and, therefore,
are subject to the waiver of liability provisions in section 1879 of the act. (See SS
343Off.)

3. *Application of Guidelines.* The following discussion illustrates the application of the above guidelines to the more common situations in which the reason-
ableness and necessity of speech services furnished is a significant issue:

a. *Restorative Therapy.* If an individual's expected restorative potential
   would be insignificant in relation to the extent and duration of speech pa-

thology services required to achieve such potential, the services would not be considered reasonable and necessary. In addition, there must be an expectation that the patient's condition will improve significantly in a reasonable (and generally predictable) period of time. If, at any point in the treatment of an illness or injury, it is determined that the expectations will not materialize, the services will no longer constitute covered speech pathology services, as they would no longer be reasonable and necessary for the treatment of the patient's condition and would be excluded from coverage under section 1862 (a) (1).

b. *Maintenance Program.* After the initial evaluation of the extent of the disorder or illness, if the restoration potential is judged insignificant or, after a reasonable period of trial, the patient's response to treatment is judged insignificant or at a plateau, an appropriate functional maintenance program may be established. The specialized knowledge and judgment of a qualified speech pathologist may be required if the treatment aim of the physician is to be achieved; e.g., a multiple sclerosis patient may require the services of a speech pathologist to establish a maintenance program designed to fit the patient's level of function. In such a situation, the initial evaluation of the patient's needs, the designing by the qualified speech pathologist of a maintenance program which is appropriate to the capacity and tolerance of the patient and the treatment objectives of the physician, the instruction of the patient and supportive personnel (e.g., aides or nursing personnel, or family members where speech pathology is being furnished on an outpatient basis) in carrying out the program, and such infrequent reevaluations as may be required, would constitute covered speech therapy. After the maintenance program has been established and instructions have been given for carrying out the program, the services of the speech pathologist would no longer be covered, as they would no longer be considered reasonable and necessary for the treatment of the patient's condition and would be excluded from coverage under section 1862 (a) (1).

If a patient has been under a restorative speech pathology program, the speech pathologist should regularly reevaluate the condition and adjust the treatment program. Consequently, during the course of treatment, the speech pathologist should determine when the patient's restorative potential will be achieved and the time frame for the restorative program required. The speech pathologist should also instruct the patient, supportive personnel, or family members in the carrying out of the program. A separate charge for the establishment of the maintenance program under these circumstances would not be recognized. Moreover, where a maintenance program is not established until after the restorative speech pathology program has been completed, it would not be considered reasonable and necessary to the treatment of the patient's condition and would be excluded from coverage under section 1862 (a) (1) since the maintenance program should have been established during the active course of treatment.

4. *Types of Services.* Speech pathology services can be grouped into two main categories: services concerned with diagnosis or evaluation and therapeutic services.

a. *Diagnostic and Evaluation Services.* Unless excluded by section 1862 (a) (7) of the law, these services are covered if they are reasonable and necessary. The speech pathologist employs a variety of formal and informal language assessment tests to ascertain the type, causal factor(s), and severity of the speech and language disorders. Reevaluation would be covered only if the patient exhibited a change in functional speech or motivation, clearing of confusion, or the remission of some other medical condition which previously contraindicated speech pathology. However, monthly reevaluations, e.g., a Porch Index of Communicative Ability (PICA) for a patient undergoing a restorative speech pathology program, are to be considered a part of the treatment session and could not be covered as a separate evaluation for billing purposes.

b. *Therapeutic Services.* The following are examples of common medical disorders and resulting communication deficits which may necessitate active restorative therapy:

(i)   Cerebrovascular disease such as cerebral vascular accidents presenting with dysphagia, aphasia/dysphasia, apraxia, and dysarthria;

(ii) Neurological disease such as Parkinsonism or Multiple Sclerosis may exhibit dysarthria, dysphagia, or inadequate respiratory volume/control;

(iii) Mental retardation with disorders such as aphasia or dysarthria; and

(iv) Laryngeal carcinoma requiring laryngectomy resulting in aphonia may warrant therapy of the laryngectomized patient so he can develop new communication skills through esophageal speech and/or use of the electrolarynx.

NOTE: Many patients who do not require speech pathology services as defined above do require services involving nondiagnostic, non-therapeutic, routing, repetitive, and reinforced procedures or services for their general good and welfare; e.g., the practicing of word drills. Such services do not constitute speech pathology services for Medicare purposes and would not be covered since they do not require performance by or the supervision of a qualified speech pathologist.

Speech-Language Pathology Adult Home Health Functional Outcome Measure

Agency/Branch _____ **MR#** _____

Date: _____ ❑ Admission ❑ Recertification (1 2 3) ❑ Discharge

Patient Name: _____ Sex: M F   D.O.B. _____/_____ /_____

Medical Dx: _____ Onset Date _____

Treatment Dx/Condition: _____

Medical HX (Hospitalization, Surgeries, Previous Tx, Current Medications, etc.):

_____

_____

Patient's primary physician _____

Physician restricted activities _____

Level of ADL/IADL function previous 12 months: ❑ Independent–Complete
❑ Independent–Partial   ❑ Dependent

Communication/cognitive abilities previous 12 months:
❑ Independent–Complete   ❑ Independent–Partial   ❑ Dependent

Psychosocial Status—Patient Lives with: ❑ Alone   ❑ Spouse
❑ Family member/caregiver   ❑ Nonfamily caregiver

Patient Lives in Home Owned by: ❑ Self   ❑ Family member
❑ Nonfamily member   ❑ Assisted living facility

Safety in Living Environment
❏ No safety hazards observed   ❏ Impaired physical ability
❏ Impaired cognition   ❏ Impaired communication   ❏ Environment
❏ Other _____

Functional Limitations:
❏ Safety   ❏ Cognition   ❏ Communication   ❏ Speech   ❏ Language
❏ Hearing   ❏ Vision   ❏ Swallowing   ❏ Mobility   ❏ ADLs/IADLs
❏ Environment   ❏ Caregiver/family actions/support
❏ Other _____

Functional Assessment

Name of Interviewee: _____
❏ Caregiver Interview   ❏ Patient Interview (when no caregiver)

	Always	Usually	Sometimes	Seldom	Never	Does therapist agree?	
Is patient's orientation or memory a problem in his/her daily routine?	❏	❏	❏	❏	❏	Yes	No
Does patient have drooling, chewing, or swallowing problems?	❏	❏	❏	❏	❏	Yes	No
Is patient able to understand information when it is communicated by others?	❏	❏	❏	❏	❏	Yes	No
Is patient able to appropriately interact with others?	❏	❏	❏	❏	❏	Yes	No

How often does patient require verbal or physical assistance with self-care? E.g., of every 4 times the patient tries, how many times does he/she need help?

	4/4	3/4	2/4	1/4	0/4 occasions		
1. Personal/Hygiene (e.g., bathing, dressing, brushing teeth)	❏	❏	❏	❏	❏	Yes	No
2. Food Purchases (e.g., grocery store activities)	❏	❏	❏	❏	❏	Yes	No
3. Meal Preparation (e.g., planning, organizing, preparing foods)	❏	❏	❏	❏	❏	Yes	No
4. Feeding (e.g., getting food/drink to mouth; sitting balance)							

	4/4	3/4	2/4	1/4	0/4 occasions
5. Household maintenance (e.g., cleaning, laundry, repairs, lawn)	❏	❏	❏	❏	❏ Yes No
6. Mobility (e.g., ability to move around w/ or w/o devices)	❏	❏	❏	❏	❏ Yes No
7. Transfers (e.g., getting out of bed/chairs, into tub, toilet)	❏	❏	❏	❏	❏ Yes No
8. Money Management (e.g., check writing/ balance, money exchange)	❏	❏	❏	❏	❏ Yes No
9. Transportation (e.g., arranging for travel; car transfers)	❏	❏	❏	❏	❏ Yes No
10. Taking medicines or following other medical or therapy instructions	❏	❏	❏	❏	❏ Yes No
11. Using a telephone (e.g., basic needs and emergency use)	❏	❏	❏	❏	❏ Yes No

Type of assistance usually provided: ❏ NA   ❏ Verbal only
❏ Physical only   ❏ Verbal and Physical   ❏ None

Caregiver perceives extra effort required to meet patient needs as being:
❏ 5–very high   ❏ 4–high   ❏ 3–somewhat high   ❏ 2–somewhat low
❏ 1–low   ❏ NA

Patient/family understanding of patient: condition: ❏ good   ❏ fair
❏ poor   needs: ❏ good   ❏ fair   ❏ poor

Other patient service needs identified: ❏ OT   ❏ PT   ❏ MSW   ❏ RN
❏ H H aide   ❏ Other _____

Patient/Caregiver goals and expectations for therapy ❏ None _____
_____
_____

Clinical findings and skilled services provided this visit: Overall degree of functional severity is: WFL   Mild   Moderate   Severe   Non-functional
_____
_____
_____
_____   ❏ End ❏ To addendum

The results of this assessment/plan of care/discharge summary were discussed with me. I understood and am in agreement with information communicated to me.

Signature of Patient/Caregiver   Date

Signature of Speech-Language Pathologist   Date

Functional Communication/Cognition Assessment

Patient Name _____ Assessment Date _____

Years of education: _____   Handedness _____

Cognition* _____ Total Score (30 max)   Must be completed each assessment

_____ 1. What is the year, month, season, date, and day? (5)
_____ 2. Where are we? State, county, town, address (4)
_____ 3. What is your birth date? (1)
_____ 4. Repeat this group of words after me: (apple, table, clock) (3)
_____ 5. Serial 7s: Count backward from 100 by 7, stop after 5
         answer OR Spell "WORLD" backward. (Give 1 point for each correct
         answer)
_____ 6. Ask to repeat the names of the three objects in #4 (3)
_____ 7. Name 2 objects: pencil (or pen) and watch (2)
_____ 8. Repeat the phrase "No ifs, ands, or buts" (1)
_____ 9. Follow the three-stage command:
         Take a paper in your right (left) hand, fold in half, put it on the floor
         (your lap) (3)
_____ 10. Read and obey the following: (1) (see p. 214)
          CLOSE YOUR EYES
_____ 11. Write a sentence (1)
_____ 12. Copy this design (1) (see p. 215)
          Maximum score 30. Score = 25–30 is benign forgetfulness; 22–24 is
          mild cognitive impairment; <22 is dementia.

Legend for Response Scoring:

Accuracy	Accurate	Accurate	Accurate	Inaccurate
Assist	No assistance	No assistance	Assisted	
Delay	< 5 sec.	> 5 < 15 sec.	<15 sec.	and/or > 15 sec.
Points	2 points	1 point	.5 point	0 point

_____

Source: "Mini Mental State: A Practical Method for Grading the Cognitive State of Patients for the Clinician." *Journal of Psychiatric Research,* 12/3): 189–198, 1975. The copyright in the Mini Mental State Examination is wholly owned by the Mini Mental LLC, a Massachusetts limited liability company. For information about how to obtain permission to use or reproduce the Mini Mental State Examination, please contact John Gonsalves Jr., Administrator of the Mini Mental LLC, at 31 St. James Avenue, Suite 1, Boston, Massachusetts, 02116, (617) 587-4215. © 1998, MMLLC.

Reasoning/Problem Solving, Sequencing, Spatial Relations
_____ Total Score (10 max) Must be completed at each assessment.

_____ 1. What does "stitch in time saves nine" mean?
_____ 2. You have forgotten how much medicine to take. Tell me how you will find that information.
(Look on the bottle, call the drugstore, call the physician/nurse)
_____ 3. Your physician has an office on the second floor of a four-story building: Describe how you will get to the second floor office when you arrive. (directory, stairs, elevator)
_____ 4. You are going to buy a gallon of milk at the grocery store. The milk will cost $2.40. You have a $5 bill. How much money should the cashier give you back?
_____ 5. You are in line at the drugstore. Another person gets in line after you do. Is that person in front of or behind you?

Comprehension/Recall/Recognition _____ Total Score (12 max)
❏ Formal reassessment is not indicated based on skilled and interview probes and performance WFLs at initial assessment.

Comprehension of gestures (4): Watch what I do and then tell me what it means.
_____ 1. Examiner nods his/her head (yes).
_____ 2. Examiner shakes his/her head (no).

Answer Yes/No questions (8):
I am going to ask you some questions; I want you to answer the questions with either yes or no as quickly as possible.
_____ 1. Does breakfast come before dinner?
_____ 2. Is a quarter worth more than a dime?
_____ 3. Is it safe to take another person's medicine?
_____ 4. Can smoke cause fire?

Patient Name _____ Assessment Date _____

Legend for Response Scoring:

Accuracy	Accurate	Accurate	Accurate	Inaccurate
Assist	No assistance	No assistance	Assisted	
Delay	< 5 sec.	> 5 < 15 sec.	<15 sec.	and/or > 15 sec.
Points	2 points	1 point	.5 point	0 point

Following commands/directives (10):
I am going to ask you to do some things for me. Just do exactly what I say as quickly as possible.

One step:	_____	1. Show me the door.
	_____	2. Make the "thumbs up" sign.
Two step:	_____	1. Turn your head and lower your chin.
	_____	2. Raise your arm and bend your elbow.
Three step:	_____	1. Bend your leg, lean forward, and push up OR Pucker your lips, puff your cheeks, and breathe out your nose.
	_____	2. See MMSE

> Expression _____ Total Score (30 + 18 for semantic fluency = 48 max)

Automatic/Responsive Speech (10):
I am going to ask you to say some things to me. Do what I ask you to do as quickly as you can.

Tell me the first word you think of when I say:
_____ 1. Hot and (cold)
_____ 2. In and (out)
_____ 3. Count to five for me.
Say exactly what I say (imitation)
_____ 5. Door-Doorknob-Doorkeeper-Dormitory
_____ 6. Indescribably delicious

Confrontation Naming—see MMSE (i.e., pen or pencil and watch)

Naming by Function (6): Tell me:
_____ 1. Something with which you can write (pen, pencil)
_____ 2. Something with which you can tell time (watch, clock)
_____ 3. Something which you might feel (tactile, emotion)

Semantic fluency task: _____ Total number of words recalled in 1 minute
In one minute, name as many foods as you can, that you would find in a supermarket. Prompt if necessary at 30 second mark with "Keep thinking of words, you still have time left." Pass with 18 food words; Fail = <18.

1.	2.	3.	4.	5.	6.	7.
8.	9.	10.	11.	12.	13.	14.
15.	16.	17.	18.	(max required)		

Verbal description (Boston) (6): _____

_____ 1. Account is relevant and organized. (5 accurate observations related to major events in picture)
_____ 2. Account is syntactically appropriate
_____ 3. Account is fluent

Pragmatics (8):
_____ 1. Appropriate conversational initiation and turn taking.
_____ 2. Able to maintain topic of conversation.
_____ 3. Communication content is socially appropriate

Reading _____ Total Score (6 max)

Read this and show it to me (reads and understands words) (see p. 216):
_____ 1. Pen
_____ 2. Watch
Read this and do what it says (reads aloud and understands sentences):
_____ 1. Lower your chin and swallow.   (2. See MMSE)

Patient Name _____ Assessment Date_____

Legend for Response Scoring:

Accuracy	Accurate	Accurate	Accurate	Inaccurate
Assist	No assistance	No assistance	Assisted	
Delay	< 5 sec.	> 5 < 15 sec.	<15 sec.	and/or > 15 sec.
Points	2 points	1 point	.5 point	0 point

Writing _____ Total Score (6 max)

_____ 1. Sign your name.

_____ 2. Write telephone number you use in emergencies [If can't do, tell to write 911 (assistance)].

_____ 3. Write something you can eat/drink. [If can't do, ask to write water (assistance)].

Dysphagia/Oral-Neuromuscular/Motor Speech Skilled Observation and Assessment

---

Legend for degree of impairment/problem:
7=WNL   6=WFL   5=Supervision   4=Mild   3=Moderate
2=Moderate to Severe   1=Severe   0=Nonfunctional
UST=Unsafe to test   DNT=did not test

Swallowing
Yes No Appropriate Positioning during Oral Intake
_____ Lip Seal: Drooling? L R   Spillage of food? L R
_____ Bolus manipulation and A-P Transit
_____ Pocketing of foods? L R
_____ Cough on demand
_____ Dry swallow on demand
_____ Clear airway/throat on demand
_____ Total

Respiration
_____ Sustained phonation (WFL ≥ 15 sec.)
_____ Breath support for swallow
_____ Breath support for speech
_____ Total
Yes No Hx of pneumonia   Yes No Hx of reflux
Yes No MBS performed _____
Yes No MBS recommended_____

Neuromuscular Assessment	ROM R L	Strength R L	MANUAL MUSCLE TEST (Daniels and Worthingham, 1986—modified) ROM: Degree of impairment (see legend above) Strength: 5=Normal (+ or –) 4=Good (+ or –) 3=Fair (+ or –) 2=Poor (+ or –) 1=Trace (+ or –) 0=Zero (0)
			Comments:
Trunk			
Head/Neck			
Mandibular			
Buccal			
Labial			
Lingual			
Palatal			
Pharyngeal/ Laryngeal			

Total   __ __ __ __

Diet stage recommended—Functional Oral Intake Scale (Crary, 1988 by permission)

_____   Level 1: No oral intake (NPO)

_____   Level 2: Tube dependent diet (Experiments inconsistently w/ small amounts of food or liquid; nutritionally dependent on tube)

_____   Level 3: Tube dependent diet (Consistently intakes certain foods/liquids by mouth; nutritionally dependent on tube)

_____   Level 4: Total diet by oral intake (Single consistency of food/liquid, eg, puree or thickened)

_____   Level 5: Total diet by oral intake (Multiple consistencies, but requires special preparation and with food/liquid restrictions)

_____   Level 6: Total diet by oral intake (No specific food preparation, but specific food limitations, eg., no meats)

_____   Level 7: Total diet by oral intake (No diet restrictions)

Diet consistencies recommended: _____

Voice and Motor Speech

Pitch	❏ WFL	❏ High	❏ Low	❏ Monotone	❏ Pitchbreak
Loudness	❏ WFL	❏ Loud	❏ Soft	❏ Monoloudness	
Quality	❏ WFL	❏ Breathy	❏ Strident	❏ Harsh	❏ Hoarse
	❏ Wet				

Apraxia: None   Mild   Moderate   Severe
Dysarthria: None   Mild   Moderate   Severe
Speech intelligibility: WFL (90%)   Mild (75%)   Moderate (60%)
                             Severe (50%)   Nonverbal (0%)

Respiration and phonation coordination: ❏ adequate   ❏ not adequate

Visual neglect?   ❏ No   ❏ Yes   ❏ L   ❏ R

Diadochokinetic rate: ❏ adequate (>10 rep/15s)   ❏ not adequate (<10 rep/15s)

Rehab Concepts™

☐ Addendum
☐ Continuation of Skilled Assessment Findings, Observations, and Recommendations

Speech-Language Pathology Assessment Scales

MR# _____

Patient name _____ (Assessment) Date _____

_____
_____
_____
_____
_____
_____
_____
_____
_____
_____
_____
_____
_____
_____
_____
_____
_____
_____
_____
_____
_____
_____
_____
_____
_____
_____
_____
_____
_____

Agency/Branch _____ Therapist's Signature _____

Speech Therapy Plan of Care/Progress Note to Physician

Patient Name: _____ M.R. #: _____
Agency SOC: _____
❑ Initial POC   ❑ Recertification (1 2 3)   ❑ Modified POC
❑ Progress Note to Physician—   30   60   day
(Re) certification period covered: from _____ to_____
Primary/Referring Physician: _____

Functional Limitations: ❑ Safety   ❑ Cognition   ❑ Communication
❑ Speech   ❑ Language   ❑ Hearing   ❑ Vision   ❑ Swallowing
❑ ADL/IADLs   ❑ Environment   ❑ Caregiver/Family Acitons/Support
❑ Mobility   ❑ Other _____

Homebound status: ❑ Bed/chairbound
❑ Requires considerable effort to leave home   ❑ Physician Restrictions
❑ Requires supervision 2nd to mental confusion to leave home
❑ Physical limitations   ❑ Other

Rehab potential ❑ is / ❑ continues to be: ❑ Good   ❑ Fair   ❑ Poor

Other needs identified: ❑ OT   ❑ PT   ❑ MSW   ❑ RN   ❑ HHA
❑ Other _____

PLAN OF CARE: Frequency and Duration _____
Anticipated Discharge Date _____
    ❑ C1–Evaluation   ❑ C7–Reserved
    ❑ C2–Voice disorders Tx   ❑ C8–Non-Oral Communication
    ❑ C3–Speech Articulation disorders Tx   ❑ C9–Pt/Cg/Family Instruction/Ed
    ❑ C4–Dysphagia Tx   ❑ C9–Cognitive disorders
    ❑ C5–Language disorders Tx   ❑ C9–Other _____
    ❑ C6–Aural Rehabilitation
Clinical pathway for _____ will be followed.   ❑ N/A

Interventions Planned: ❑ Reduce Impairment
❑ Teach Compensatory Techniques/Strategies
❑ Substitute/Change Activity   ❑ Assistive Technology
❑ Use of Assistance of Another Person   ❑ Other _____
Safety Training to Include: _____
Required Supplies and Equipment:_____

Short Term Objectives to be achieved in _____ weeks
Objective 1: _____
Objective 2: _____
Objective 3: _____
Objective 4: _____
Objective 5: _____

Functional Long Term Goals to be achieved in _____ ❑ weeks/ ❑ months
Goal 1: _____
Goal 2: _____
Goal 3: _____
Goal 4: _____
Goal 5: _____

Patient/Family Involvement: ❑ Participated
❑ Declined to participate, but consented to therapy
❑ Declined to participate and refused therapy
Progress towards long-term goals include: ❑ Not Applicable
Goal 1: _____
Goal 2: _____
Goal 3: _____
Goal 4: _____
Goal 5: _____

Discharge Plan: Patient will be discharged from ST services when:
❑ patient achieves optimal outcome from treatment
❑ when the patient is no longer home bound   ❑ at physician request   AND
❑ to care of physician and   ❑ self   ❑ family   ❑ facility_____
❑ Other _____
Agency Communication/Conferencing: _____
_____

Therapist Signature _____ Date _____
Contract Agency _____

Physician Signature_____ Date _____
Time: _____ am pm

Close your eyes

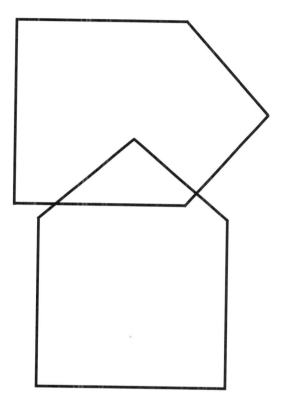

Pen

Watch

Lower your chin and swallow

CHAPTER 8

Professional Accountability through Continuous Quality Improvement

INTRODUCTION

Today, health care professionals use concepts that were once within the exclusive purview of manufacturing and other industries. Concepts such as continuous quality improvement (CQI), statistical process control, and total quality management (TQM) are emerging as the new frontier for the quality discipline. Quality in home care of tomorrow will be a process that starts when the phone rings with an inquiry and continues long after the patient is discharged. New quality assessment tools are being developed, such as outcome-based quality improvement (OBQI; e.g., the Outcome and Assessment Information Set [OASIS]), to better define the impact care has on patients' health. In addition, quality will incorporate the expectations of all customers, not just payers, as seen in the development of critical pathways. Quality will be expanded into every phase of operations and will become an integral part of the overall business plan. Quality will become synonymous with customer satisfaction, outcomes, and competency and will be the primary responsibility of a chief executive officer. It will move from the clinician's office to the boardroom.

This progressive movement of quality will be propelled by an increasingly knowledgeable consumer and fueled by regulatory and environmental mandates. Competitive advantage will drive this movement, and its parade will be national recognition. CQI will provide the foundation on which an agency can build an integrated quality program through which great achievement can be made.

Speech-language pathologists in home health care provide a unique practice, and they can have a unique role in quality improvement and management as well. The use of CQI tools in home health care will vary widely, depending on the size and complexity of the organization. For example, the CQI program of a hospital-affiliated home health agency may be organized throughout the hospital through the hospital quality management department, or it may have its own designated director or department. In many free-standing community-based agencies, the CQI functions may be incorporated into one or several existing positions. Along with the variations, however, there are similarities in all settings relative to the role of the speech-language pathologist and home health care quality assessment.

Agencies are one of the driving forces behind the move toward quality management, but speech-language pathologists should also recognize its advantages. They have an opportunity to turn quality management into a process that can work for speech-language pathology services. Since it costs less to provide quality care the first time, why not determine the right way to do something and be able to do it right the first time, and every time?

In addition, in the current environment of competition among home health providers, quality of care—and the clear proof of that quality—becomes a significant determining factor in the selection of a home health care provider. As patients become more aware of their rights and responsibilities in relation to the selection of their home health care provider, health care providers will no longer be able to rely on established referral sources. Home care organizations are having to earn the right to receive referrals, and they therefore must produce a high-quality outcome at a minimum cost. With this in mind, the clinician should consider the following components of quality:

> Quality is a long, ongoing process. To succeed, hospice and home care organizations can use information from both quality assurance and quality improvement efforts. Quality is a channel that takes time and must be done one step at a time throughout all levels of an organization within the confines of the restrictive legislative environment. A commitment to quality pays off, as many success stories in the health-care field demonstrate—it is a process that benefits the entire organization and the patients it serves. From a financial perspective, quality could "save your hide." From the regulatory perspective, quality is not just a good idea anymore—it's the law. (Joint Commission on Accreditation of Healthcare Organizations [the Joint Commission], 1993, p. 91)

Speech-language pathologists who practice in home health care need to be familiar with quality assessment, its concepts, and its terms so that they may more effectively participate in quality assessment procedures. Through this participation, speech-language pathologists can ensure, in a measurable, scientific manner, that their services are effective, while educating others on the services that speech-language pathology has to offer. Participating in the process of assessing quality ensures the profession's place in the health care community of providers.

This chapter is not intended to comprehensively cover quality assessment in home health care today. The chapter provides an overview of major aspects of

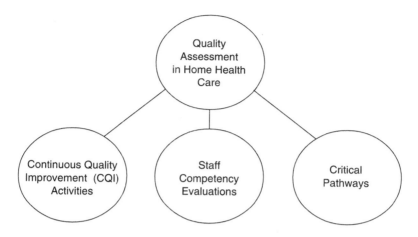

Figure 8–1 Quality Assessment Initiatives in Home Health Care

quality assessment currently being used and also examines some future trends that will affect the practice of speech-language pathology in home care. The areas that are discussed in this chapter are CQI, OBQI, clinical competency, and patient outcome measures. Figure 8–1 depicts the current trends in quality assessment initiatives in home health care, which are areas important for the speech-language pathologist to know. The chapter particularly emphasizes CQI, since this form of quality assessment is the most widely used and the most well understood. Although patient outcomes, OBQI, and competencies are in the near future, their significance for the practice of speech-language pathology is not clear.

QUALITY ASSESSMENT/IMPROVEMENT: AN OVERVIEW

Harris (1997) discusses *quality assurance (QA)* as a term that has been heard frequently in home health care. She discusses what QA means and how it is accomplished. The *Taber's Cyclopedic Medical Dictionary* (1989) defines *quality* as "a character with respect to excellence, fineness, or grade of excellence." *Assurance* is defined as "the understanding or making of certain: a positive declaration intended to give confidence." By combining these two definitions then, Harris says that QA can be defined as the process of making certain or guaranteeing that high-quality care will be provided to patients, which will instill confidence in the product or services provided.

A QA program is designed to demonstrate and mark the degree to which an organization's actual performance compares with expected outcomes (Gould & Ruane, 1988). A QA program in a home health agency is necessary for multiple reasons: to monitor and evaluate patient care; to identify, hire, and retain the appropriate level of personnel to meet patient needs; to meet standards established by Medicare Conditions of Participation, accrediting bodies, professional organizations, and the agency itself; to address risk management issues; and to address and resolve identified problems.

CONTINUOUS QUALITY IMPROVEMENT

The statistical tools for improving quality came to the health care industry from the manufacturing environment, where these methods were tested and found to be the key to sustained improvements. The following are some basic concepts of CQI (Harris, 1994):

- Every problem has a root cause based in either a system or a process.
- Every process (or system) has a distinct organizational flow and specified decision points for alternative actions or behaviors.
- Every process in health care, either clinical or administrative, has an upstream and a downstream customer who will determine quality at the point of interface.
- Every process generates or produces some output that can be either measured or counted.
- Every process has a pattern or shape that is discernible when viewed in graphic form. This shape becomes the basis for all statistical studies in the improvement efforts and is commonly referred to as the *bell-shaped curve*.
- Every process will have variation. Variation is a natural state but is the enemy of quality.

The Quality Improvement Model for Home Care

Previously, quality had a generic definition. However, traditional thinking about concepts of quality no longer applies in today's highly competitive marketplace in which home care agencies and speech-language pathologists contract for services. In the past, quality was considered only a clinical function, and management delegated the assurance of quality to a director or a QA committee. However, the days when quality was "assumed" are long gone. Today TQM is about doing business. It must be management led and customer oriented. Total quality is not just the latest management fad; it is a new way of thinking that will require fundamental changes in the way home health agencies and contracting speech-language pathologists will do business. Regardless of whether speech-language pathologists are independent contractors or employees of the home health agency, it is important for them to know the basics of TQM as seen in today's home health care arena. Staff (both contract and agency personnel) must know the requirements or expectations of their roles, and have them in written form, if they are to meet those expectations. It is incumbent upon speech-language pathologists to obtain QA programs from each agency with which they work. The more aware the speech-language pathologist becomes of written expectations, the better are the chances for improved performance that improves patient care outcomes. In fact, the meaning behind CQI is a continuous improvement in process and requirements to better meet customer expectations. Process cannot be improved without a definition of the process or without clear written instructions about the requirements. Part of this definition would be the four major components of quality care (Harris, 1994):

1. professional performance
2. efficient use of resources
3. minimal risk to the patient of injury or illness associated with care
4. patient satisfaction

Each of these components can be found in an agency's quality productivity model. The agency's model should associate quality care with efficiency and productivity. In fact, quality is synonymous with efficiency and productivity, for each is less effective without the other. Therefore, any agency model should begin the process of quality with written controls that assist both the managers and the employees or contractors to understand the expectations.

Quality control can be defined as a measurable process that is stated in written terms, usually as a policy and procedure of an agency, and that is derived from the expectations of customers. The policies and procedures are a basic first step in ensuring quality, since they set forth expected behavior in conformance with stated customer expectations. Davis (1994) states that policies and procedures should be written in a format that clearly defines how the procedure is to be implemented. These procedures also should include the practice or protocol of the agency for a specific function.

It is important for the speech-language pathologist to know that quality control is a proactive process whereby all the rules that must be followed are incorporated into a written measurable format and taught to those who render the care. Teaching caregivers is as important as committing the rules and regulations to paper. The best policies and procedures have little benefit if those rendering care do not know the information contained in them. Staff development is the key ingredient to successful internalization of the quality control standards, and speech-language pathologists must obtain information regarding agencies' policies and procedures for the care of patients who require the skills of a speech-language pathologist.

Quality Assurance Process

Quality assurance is a standard by which the measurable process specified in quality control is validated. In other words, QA is a retroactive monitoring process. Like most audits, QA is performed after the fact. Audit results can be evaluated to determine whether standards were met. There are a number of different QA audits or surveillance tools used by agencies. Because of the variety of audits and the time needed to go through the audit process, it is important that speech-language pathologists know the priorities of the agencies and the tools that they wish to use for QA and surveillance activities in order of importance or impact on patient care outcomes. The outcomes expected should be stated as measures of performance (thresholds).

The many varieties of QA audit tools can be grouped into the following types (Davis, 1994):

- *Quality assurance:* An audit process by which professional practice is validated using nationally recognized standards of care by diagnosis or disease state.
- *Utilization review:* An audit process by which appropriate utilization of services, including efficient use of resources and visits, is validated in accordance with guidelines established by payer source.
- *Field review:* An audit process by which appropriate clinical technique is validated on the basis of standards of care in the home setting.
- *Administrative review:* An audit process by which the clinical record, optimal processes, or both are validated in accordance with established policies and procedures of the agency.

The aforementioned types of audits are used as a standard in most agencies in some form. Another type of auditing information, skills validation for all patient caregivers, is not revealed in most of the literature but is now an important part of the Joint Commission's accreditation standards for home health. The Joint Commission requires that the clinical skills of each patient care provider be evaluated annually. Appendix 8–A shows an example of a clinical skills validation checklist.

Quality Continuation

The next phase in the quality system is quality continuation. Quality continuation is proactive and deals exclusively with constant self-measurement by known standards. The known standards usually come from the specifiers under the quality control program as taught to and reinforced with clinical staff and administration. Quality continuation then is the allotment of quality policy, procedure, practice, hiring criteria, training, rewards, and recognition.

Quality Improvement

The fourth and final phase of quality management is quality improvement. This phase is the sum total of all the other components and is the goal of all agencies.

Davis (1994) states that quality improvement does not just happen. It is the end result of developing the standards, implementing the QA activities, and continuing to build quality by staff development. Improvement can be both proactive and retroactive, according to Davis. Quality is a never-constant, ever-changing target; therefore, changes are frequent. The health care field is in constant change, and speech-language pathologists must be prepared to keep pace with technology. The key to success is to stay high on the learning curve throughout one's professional career.

The bottom line in quality management is that customers must be satisfied with the care they receive or they will not have a perception of quality, regardless of whether all standards were in compliance. In other words, there is a difference between quality by perception and quality by fact. Speech-language pathologists should be aware that most patients and their families or caregivers do not know if the care or a procedure was technically correct. Their decision about quality depends mostly on their perception of the caregiver during the treatment interaction.

QUALITY DEFINITIONS

Speech-language pathologists should be familiar with the terminology of quality management used by their agencies. The following are some of the more common quality management terms and definitions.

Doing the Right Thing

Efficacy: The efficacy of a procedure or treatment in relation to the patient's condition is the degree to which the care/intervention for the patient has been shown to accomplish the desired/projected outcomes.

Appropriateness: The appropriateness of a specific test, procedure, or service to meet the patient's needs is the degree to which the care/intervention provided is relevant to the patient's clinical needs, given the current state of knowledge.

Doing the Right Thing Well

Availability: The availability of the needed test, procedure, treatment, or service to the patient who needs it is the degree to which appropriate care/intervention is available to meet the patient's needs.

Timeliness: The timeliness with which a needed test, procedure, treatment, or service is provided to the patient is the degree to which the care/intervention is provided to the patient at the most beneficial or necessary time.

Effectiveness: The effectiveness with which tests, procedures, treatments, and services are provided is the degree to which the care/intervention is provided in the correct manner, given the current state of knowledge, in order to achieve the desired/projected outcome for the patient.

Continuity: The continuity of the services provided to the patient with respect to other services, practitioners, and providers and over time is the degree to which the care/intervention for the patient is coordinated among practitioners, organizations, and over time.

Safety: The safety of the patient (and others) to whom the services are provided is the degree to which the risk of an intervention and the risk in the care environment are reduced for the patient and others, including the home health provider.

Efficiency: The efficiency with which services are provided is the relationship between the outcomes (results of care) and the resources used to deliver patient care.

Respect and caring: The respect and caring with which services are provided are the degree to which the patient or a designated individual is involved in his or her own care decisions and to which those providing services do so with sensitivity and respect for the patient's needs, expectations, and individual differences.

(The Joint Commission, 1996, Section 2, p. 2)

These definitions reach to the core of performance for speech-language pathology in a home health care setting. The terminology is very useful in focusing documentation to demonstrate the need for speech-language pathology services and the value of services provided.

METHODOLOGY

Once clinicians understand quality management issues and the rationale for quality management in home health care, as discussed in the preceding, what do they do with this information? How do they use it? There are no magical formulas or cookbooks to answer these questions or that will work for all agencies for which the speech-language pathologist will work. However, there are some commonalities and essential components to consider. The speech-language pathologist must focus on the key functions that involve the provision of services within an organization's framework, keeping in mind the definitions in the preceding section as they relate to speech-language pathology services.

Although monitoring may be new to some practitioners, the concepts are basic to quality issues in home health. Practitioners may be able to add monitoring activities to their existing activity with the agency by using patient satisfaction surveys, interdisciplinary tracking of timeliness and completion of documentation, or even QA audits.

The following examples highlight some areas of monitoring to consider:

- Treatment plan is appropriate, and goals and objectives are coordinated.
- Interdisciplinary team members are involved in rehabilitation care planning.
- Evaluations are completed within 48 hours.
- Tests administered were appropriate.
- Infection control policies and procedures are followed.
- Interventions are appropriate for patient's level of functioning.

In addition to the preceding examples, the speech-language pathologist should consider some of the following areas:

- efficacy of treatment
- appropriateness of level of care or service
- family's and/or significant others' participation in discharge planning
- all communication among treatment team members
- standards for documentation within the organization and the local regulatory agencies

Components of a Complete Quality Management Program

Generally, a complete quality management program requires both quality evaluation (or QA) and aspects of both risk management and utilization review. In short, quality management interrelates with all other essential functions of a home health agency. Also, because patients are now discharged from hospitals earlier in their care process and with much more complex procedures than ever before, the clinician faces significantly increased risk. Multiskills training thus becomes essential, and basic medical procedures must be understood and demonstrated by the speech-language pathologist. Quality aspects of care might include not only procedures relating to patients with speech-language-swallowing or hearing disorders but also the speech-language pathologist's ability to handle medical situations in the home.

Continuous Quality Improvement Activities

The following CQI activities are some examples of monitoring areas that a clinician might encounter in a home health agency. This list is by no means complete and should be used only as an example.

- employee accidents/incidents
- patient accidents/incidents
- customer complaints/concerns

- customer satisfaction surveys
- medical records review

Medical Records Review

In a medical records review audit, the agency typically takes a sampling of both active and inactive records. The records are then reviewed according to established agency criteria. The persons allowed to review these records vary from agency to agency, but usually nurses and/or nursing support personnel do the review. The review process is an excellent place to start in understanding the quality management system of any agency. By sitting in on the review, clinicians can get a better understanding of the criteria with which the agency will evaluate their charts.

Patient Accidents/Incidents and Infection Tracking

Safety of patients and caregivers has become of major concern for all programs. Most agencies track all accidents and incidents relating to patients and their employees. In most cases, an agency will require the reporting of both witnessed and unwitnessed occurrences. In addition, a patient/clinician infection and exposure log is also kept. Exhibit 8–1 depicts a typical type of tracking log found in a home health agency. The report is detailed enough to track all of the occurrences. Although speech-language pathologists may be independent contractors, they still have the obligation to report these occurrences.

Customer Complaint/Concern Report

Accrediting bodies require agencies to keep a log of patient, physician, and employee complaints. These complaints are logged in the order taken. Follow-up and resolution of all entries are usually documented on the report. Some agencies have a separate form for each occurrence. Exhibit 8–2 is an example of a customer complaint/concern log.

Customer Satisfaction Surveys

Surveys are an integral part of any quality management program. Surveys assist an agency to get anonymous feedback from their customer base. Most accrediting bodies for home health require that some kind of customer surveys be completed. Agency customers include patients and their families, internal customers (e.g., agency employees), physicians, hospitals, and other entities with which the agency does business. The following are just a few examples of some surveys an agency might use.

Patient Satisfaction Survey. Patient satisfaction surveys are usually given to patients after they have been discharged from the agency. The survey might be

Exhibit 8–1 Patient Accident/Incident and Infection Tracking Log

Patient Medical Record Number	Date	Accident/Incident Codes (Type and Location)	Witnessed = W Unwitnessed = U (If witnessed, was report filed?)	Infection Name and ICD-9 Code	Staff Contacts with Methicillin-Resistant *Staphylococcus aureus* (MRSA) or Tuberculosis (TB) Patients (For 10 Days Prior to Diagnosis)	Physician Name
Trends Noted:			Total Witnessed: Total Unwitnessed:	Total Infections:	Follow-Up (If applicable):	

Exhibit 8-2 Patient Complaint/Concern Log

Note: This log should be used to record patient complaints/concerns relative to delivery of care ONLY.

Date/Time Received	Medical Record Number	ID# and Initials of Staff Receiving Complaint	Complaint Code (Code all that apply)	Discipline Code of Staff Involved in Complaint	Actions/Resolutions/Comments

general in nature or specific to a particular discipline. Usually the discipline that discharges the patient leaves the survey with the patient or family, and it is to be mailed back. Some agencies mail the survey after discharge. In any case, the survey serves as the data source for patient satisfaction. Exhibit 8–3 is an example of a patient satisfaction survey designed specifically for speech-language pathology services.

Agency Questionnaire. Many home health agencies contract to provide home health services for health care facilities. For example, an agency might contract with a skilled nursing facility or hospital for home health. In that instance, the agency would need to evaluate the facility's perception of the care the agency delivers.

Employee Satisfaction Survey. Many agencies like to see how well they are doing from an internal standpoint. Employee satisfaction surveys take many forms, including suggestion boxes, questionnaires, or even small focus groups.

Assessment of Care

How does an agency assess the care it provides to patients? At best it is a difficult task. Several assessments are generally used to determine if appropriate care is being provided. Typically, assessment of care takes the form of chart audits, routine patient staffings, and supervisory visits made with field staff. A percentage of each staff member's case charts, both active and inactive, are usually examined by an audit team. The audit team can be made up of nurses, therapists, physicians, or any combination.

Indicator Studies

Indicators identify processes, clinical events, outcomes, or areas of service and are used to examine quality-of-care issues. The three types of indicator studies are structure, process, and outcome:

- Structural studies include areas not directly associated with the actual process of care delivery.
- Process studies examine what the health care provider does to, for, and with the patient.
- Outcome studies focus on what happens to the patient as a result of the care rendered.

Most agencies have a procedure for developing indicators and determining the type of indicator study to conduct. The following is an example of the steps an agency might take in indicator development.

Exhibit 8–3 Patient Satisfaction Survey

In order to better serve you and our other patients, we need to know your evaluation of the care we provide. Please complete this survey using the following measures:

A=ALWAYS   B=USUALLY   C=SOMETIMES   D=SELDOM   E=NEVER

Was the therapist courteous and helpful?	A B C D E
Did the therapist present him- or herself in a professional manner?	A B C D E
Did the therapist appear concerned and interested in the patient/family?	A B C D E
Did the therapist inform you of your rights as a patient, and was a copy of your patient rights left with you and/or your family?	YES NO
Were the results of the evaluation, nature of the problem, and treatment plan discussed with you and your family?	YES NO
Were you involved in the planning, decision making, implementation, and evaluation of the services you were receiving?	YES NO
Were all of your questions and concerns regarding treatment or your condition answered thoroughly?	YES NO
Were you given an opportunity to be involved in setting treatment goals and/or assisting in treatment?	YES NO
Were you kept informed about progress in treatment?	A B C D E
Do you feel that the therapist spent enough time each visit?	A B C D E
Did the therapist call to schedule your initial visit?	YES NO
Were you informed of changes in the therapist's schedule and/or changes in the therapist providing treatment?	A B C D E
Do you think that therapy has enhanced your independence, self-sufficiency, and productivity?	A B C D E
Do you think that therapy has made a positive difference in your ability to function in activities of daily living?	A B C D E
Did you receive a copy of a home program?	YES NO
Please list therapy services you received:	

1. *Identify scope of service:* Indicator studies are usually based on the organization's scope of services. The typical scope of services for a home health agency includes nursing, home health aide services, therapy services, and social work. Some agencies also provide hospice care, intravenous therapy home ser-

vices, and homemaker services. Indicator studies must be process or outcome oriented.

2. *Identify the aspect of care:* Aspects of care are the immediate basis for indicator development and represent the activities with the greatest impact on the quality of patient care. The aspects of care may be based on areas of patient care delivery that are high volume, high risk, and/or problem prone.

3. *Write the indicator statement:* The indicator statement should be a short, simple, and direct statement of an activity, a process, or a procedure that should occur. It should be measurable and objective and reflect an impact on patient outcomes. For example, "Each speech-language pathologist will complete initial evaluations within 48 hours of patient admission 95 percent of the time."

4. *Identify the threshold or trigger level:* The quality management team or committee usually determines what realistic level of performance will be acceptable, measured as a percentage. In determining thresholds, the team must consider that some variables are beyond control and may prevent the indicator from occurring. Thresholds of less than 80 percent should be avoided. The threshold is the basis for measurement and comparison.

5. *Design the methodology:* The methodology is usually determined by the quality management team or committee. It is the process that will be used to determine and measure the activity. Methods must be agreed upon by the team or committee and followed uniformly by staff.

Responsibility

Who then is responsible for all of the data? In small agencies, there is usually a small committee who gathers the data and reports the information to administration. In large agencies where there are subunits or multiple sites, each subunit is responsible for its own activities, although the procedure and data collection are the same.

OUTCOME-BASED QUALITY IMPROVEMENT

Home health care represents one component of the health care continuum. The largest single component of home health care comprises services covered by Medicare. This component of Medicare has been growing rapidly, and concerns with both the cost and the quality of home care have increased along with Medicare expenditures. According to Shaughnessy and Crisler (1995), between 1990 and 1995 the number of Medicare beneficiaries receiving home health care almost doubled (from 1.9 million to 3.6 million), and annual visits per person served grew equally dramatically (from 36 to 70). The cumulative effect was to increase total Medicare home health visits from 70 million to 252 million and Medicare home health expenditures from \$3.9 billion to \$16.0 billion (Prospective Payment Assessment Commission, 1996).

As home health care visits and expenditures grow, the importance of objectively assessing the impact of care increases correspondingly. Payers are interested in the quality of care received relative to what is being paid. Although quality of health care can be examined from the perspective of structure, process, or outcomes, payers increasingly emphasize the outcomes of care, that is, what happens to a patient's health status as a result of receiving care. In addition, accreditation and certification programs, as well as state and federal government certification agencies, have become progressively more outcome oriented. Equally important, home care agencies are increasingly concerned with measuring their own performance relative to standards or the performance of other providers. This combination of factors has fueled a powerful movement toward outcome measurement in home health care.

The research that led to the development of the OBQI approach was developed for home health care nearly a decade ago with several million dollars in funding from the federal government. The resulting outcome measures system and its application for performance improvement constitute a methodology termed *outcome-based quality improvement* (OBQI) in home care. The outcome measures system was developed predominantly for Medicare beneficiaries. The resulting measures pertain to all adult patients; however, measures for younger populations, as well as specific subgroups of patients, can be developed in the future.

The focus of the OBQI approach is patient outcomes that occur over a home health care episode. The purpose of the original research was to develop valid and reliable measures of patient outcomes that could be precisely quantified and compared across home health agencies and patients.

The evolution of the outcome measures system and the performance improvement approach based on the system has involved a number of separate but integrated activities (Shaughnessy, 1991; Shaughnessy et al., 1994, 1995, 1996). They have included reviews of outcome measures and related papers, documents, and articles published in the research literature and the provider and clinical literature, as well as reviews of outcome measures being used and under development by individual agencies or groups of agencies.

The fundamental definition of a patient-level outcome is a change in health status between two or more time points. In the current OBQI system, this is the basic or anchoring definition of an outcome. It is termed an *end-result outcome* because it reflects the change in patient health status over the course of time, which is the focal point of providing health care. The two time points that are typically used to gauge outcomes in home health care are the start of care and discharge. Health status is broadly defined, encompassing physiological, functional, cognitive, mental, and social health. Illustrations of an end-result outcome include improvement in the ability to ambulate between admission and discharge, decline in dysphagia between admission and 120 days after admission, stabilization or no change in pain interfering with activities between 60 and 180 days, and improvement in ability to manage oral medications between admission and discharge.

To date, agencies and practitioners are unsure of the ramifications of the Health Care Financing Administration (HCFA) initiative in OBQI. Agencies and clinicians alike are struggling to predict the implication for their operations. To understand OBQI and the HCFA initiative, clinicians must first understand the terminology. The following describes terms that the clinician should know.

OBQI: OBQI stands for outcome-based quality improvement. The concept is the result of a research project conducted by the Center of Health Policy and Services Research in Denver and funded by the HCFA and the Robert Wood Johnson Foundation. The Omnibus Budget Reconciliation Act (OBRA) of 1987 mandated that the survey focus on outcomes of care. The directive led to the HCFA's Home Health Initiative, which will include two significant components: (1) a complete revision of the Conditions of Participation, focusing on outcomes, and (2) OBQI, a future requirement of Medicare certification. The HCFA will require agencies to monitor their performance through key outcome measures and to implement a program to improve care.

Outcome: An outcome is the result of care, in other words, what actually happened to the patient. OBQI reflects the shift in health care emphasis from processes (how something is done) to outcomes (the results of what has been done). Patients and payers want favorable outcomes from home health care. Accreditation programs have become more outcome focused in their standards and evaluation processes.

Outcome Measure: An outcome measure is a quantification of a change in health status between two or more moments in time. This change can be positive (the patient improves), neutral (the patient stabilizes), or negative (the patient deteriorates). The ability to measure outcomes will be crucial to OBQI.

Medicare OASIS: OASIS stands for the Outcome and Assessment Information Set that the HCFA is proposing for the purposes of OBQI under Medicare and as part of the new Conditions of Participation. The OASIS data set will be the basis of outcome measurement. The data set consists of more than 70 data elements and provides a structured approach to patient assessment. The OASIS data set will minimize the subjectivity and variations in the process of assessing a patient's abilities. It also provides the basis for consistent measurement of outcomes over time. The following is an example:

> An agency's assessment instrument evaluates the patient's ambulatory ability simply, using three choices: independent, partially independent, or dependent. The OASIS data set includes five well-defined steps for assessment of ambulation, ranging from bedfast, unable to be up in a

chair, to able to independently work on even or uneven surfaces and climb stairs with or without railing.

Two-Stage CQI Screen: One of the OBQI fundamentals is that patient outcomes should be the focus of the documentation of expected outcomes. Emphasis will be on review and updating of patient goals and evaluating patient progress toward goals.

In summary, OBQI presents an interesting arena for the speech-language pathologist. No longer will clinicians be able to establish vague goals (e.g., the patient will improve his ability to swallow). They will be required to document the effectiveness of their treatment in improving the patient's health. The next section addresses how the clinician can attempt to meet these requirements by development of critical pathways.

CRITICAL PATHWAYS

Enormous and rapid changes in the delivery of traditional health care services have occurred over the last decade. With alterations in the fabric of provider payment, the rise in health care costs, and innovations in medical technology, successful patient care as a defensive strategy to control costs is imperative. Case management and managed care have emerged as cost-effective designs specifically aimed at obtaining desired patient outcomes (Bower, 1992). Early evidence suggests that the critical pathway, introduced as the tool to enhance managed care, can significantly improve multidisciplinary communications and coordination of patient activities in addition to controlling costs.

Derived from a term in computer technology, the critical pathway identifies a particular progression of events, which may include physician orders and multidisciplinary standards of practice. Each step in the pathway process must be completed in sequence before the next step is undertaken. A deviation is a variance or detour from the pathway that increases the period and/or visits allotted to achieve specific goals.

Because pathways focus on sites of care and/or timeliness, the number of days, weeks, or visits generally represents effective measurements to gauge the outcome of care rendered. Pathways will differ, because patient protocols and physician orders vary greatly. The speech-language pathologist should view the pathway as a unique version of the care plan that incorporates standing orders (Zander, 1988). Experts in the nursing field recommend that agencies include the pathway form as part of the permanent medical record.

High-volume cases lend themselves well to pathway development. One specific diagnosis should be chosen to begin the process. Figure 8–2 is a model that has been useful in implementing the use of critical pathways. Initially, staff should review a sample of cases to decide which particular cases occurred most frequently, which speech-language pathology interventions occurred most frequently, and when these interventions occurred during care. Then staff must develop time frames, interventions, and expected patient outcomes for the pathway after careful case and record review. The pathway should contain realistic goals

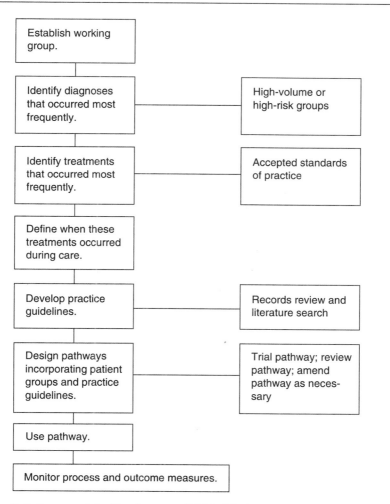

Figure 8–2 Framework for Development of Critical Pathways

and interventions and reflect care that is specific to the practice of speech-language pathology.

Critical pathways are grids that depict patient and staff behavior against a timeline for a specific patient population. When expected patient outcomes do not occur within the time frame prescribed, variances result. Positive variances occur when patients progress toward outcomes faster than anticipated. Negative variances occur when there is a time delay in attaining patient outcomes (Zander, 1993). Zander (1989) developed three broad categories to classify variances according to causality, as follows:

1. variances caused within the system
2. variances caused by the practitioner
3. variances caused by the patient

Most home health agencies already have CQI activities in place. These three variance groupings help an agency identify problems and refine processes needed to improve quality. Variances caused by the system describe pathway detours directly related to agency system problems. These variances are most commonly found in the acute care setting. An example of a home care system variance is a nurse not performing wound care within the specified visits as a result of tardy delivery of supplies. The variance investigation by the clinician later reveals that the supply company is mailing soft goods instead of driving them to patients' homes. Tracking to provide early identification of these kinds of problems can allow the agency to promptly correct them.

Because of the nature of patient care in the home, variances caused by clinicians are also common in the home health setting. For example, a patient newly diagnosed as diabetic is to have a blood sample drawn by the nurse for glucose analysis during the first week of service. This activity is inadvertently omitted by a practitioner, and the patient's dosage of insulin is not adjusted correctly. The practitioner has created a delay in the desired patient outcomes by not following the plan of care.

Patient variances relate directly to the patient; that is, the failure to meet the timeline for expected patient outcomes is due solely to patient variables. For example, a patient with acquired immune deficiency syndrome requires teaching about symptom control on the third visit. The nurse is unable to instruct the patient because of pain-management problems. The patient's uncontrolled pain creates a delay on the pathway. Patient variances most commonly occur in the community health setting.

Analysis of pathway variance is essential to improving the quality of service that the agency and/or specific disciplines offer. Variance reviews should occur, at a minimum, at the end of each month and at the time of recertification or discharge. The clinician records the variance on a tracking sheet while concurrently noting in the progress note the patient outcomes due to treatment (Zander, 1993).

Sample Pathway

A sample critical pathway for a home care patient with dysphagia is presented in Exhibit 8–4. Because the clinical staff that developed the tool found that 80 percent of patients with dysphagia require 24 visits of service, that time frame is used. Exhibit 8–5 is an example of a variance tracking tool. The tracking form highlights the data that speech-language pathologists need to collect to improve quality.

Speech-language pathologists should base their pathways on practices, policies, and procedures specific to the agencies they serve and the population they treat. In both the exhibits presented, the clinician will note the overall pathway to be followed. In most pathways, practitioners indicate a day-by-day process. However, the focus group that developed this pathway decided that patient response in rehabilitation is too variable on each visit and therefore developed end-result outcomes with expected time frames and/or visits for the outcomes to be achieved.

Benefits of Critical Pathways

According to Bower (1992), the critical pathway stimulates the creation of new or refined services. Generally, pathways also increase interdisciplinary referrals and more appropriate utilization of staff other than nursing.

When the pathway is reviewed with the patient and family, they tend to improve their self-care capabilities and increase their adherence to therapeutic programs. The patient is an active participant in the care plan, which also meets federal and accreditation criteria. Finally, the pathway improves patient satisfaction. By discussing expectations of service on the first visit, the speech-language pathologist gives the patient the opportunity to verbalize concerns about the care before interventions take place.

Conservation of the clinician's time is an indirect benefit of critical pathway use. The tool is easy for staff to follow, helps prevent redundancy of service, and provides for shorter, more efficient reports. The pathway can replace all or part of the care plan, daily notes, and update reports, thereby streamlining documentation.

Rationale

Speech-language pathologists need to continue to develop and expand their pathways to include all aspects of care rendered to the patients they treat so that

Exhibit 8–4 Critical Pathway: Dysphagia

Name: _____   Agency: _____   Social Security Number: _____

Skilled Service	Admission Visit	Home Education	Expected Outcome	Achieved Y N NA	Date

NURSING:
Expected Number of Visits: 9
	❏ Obtain history and physical
	❏ Assess vital signs
	❏ Assess lung sounds
	❏ Assess nutritional intake
	❏ Assess skin color
	❏ Assess effectiveness of meds
	INSTRUCTION
	  ❏ Patient rights
	  ❏ Financial liability for care
	  ❏ Home safety
	  ❏ Use of pathway
	  ❏ Medication regimen
		Instruct patient and caregiver in and establish home program for nutrition, medication compliance, home safety and reinforce dysphagia program	Improved nutritional intake, compliance with medications, stabilized medical condition		

SPEECH-LANGUAGE PATHOLOGY Expected Number of Visits: 24	❏ Assess swallowing per bedside evaluation ❏ May recommend an instrumental assessment ❏ Assess cognitive abilities	Instruct patient and caregiver in and establish home program for: ❏ diet consistency	Improved neuromuscular control of the swallowing structures for safe swallowing of the appropriate diet		

continues

Exhibit 8–4 continued

Name: _____ Agency: _____ Social Security Number: _____

Skilled Service	Admission Visit	Home Education	Expected Outcome	Achieved Y N NA	Date
	❏ Assess patient and caregiver ability to carry out home dysphagia program ❏ Discuss dysphagia home safety program and leave copy in the home ❏ Instruct in use of pathway ❏ Discuss plan of care ❏ Implement discharge planning	❏ safe swallow strategies ❏ appropriate cueing to assist patient in safe swallowing ❏ neuromuscular reeducation ❏ safe swallowing maneuvers	consistency, de-creased risk for aspiration, patient able to demonstrate safe swallowing maneuvers		
OCCUPA-TIONAL THERAPY Expected Number of Visits: 6	❏ Perform initial evaluation for upper extremity strength and feeding program ❏ Follow all precautions ❏ Discuss expectations of program	Instruct patient and caregiver in and establish a home program for feeding and upper extremity strengthening	Patient will exhibit upper extremity strength sufficient to carry out a feeding program.		

continues

Exhibit 8–4 continued

Name: _____   Agency: _____   Social Security Number: _____

Skilled Service	Admission Visit	Home Education	Expected Outcome	Achieved Y N NA	Date
PHYSICAL THERAPY Expected Number of Visits: 6	❏ Perform initial assessment for positioning and trunk stability ❏ Follow all precautions ❏ Discuss expectations of positioning and trunk program	Instruct patient and caregiver in and establish home program for positioning and trunk stability	Improved positioning and trunk stability for swallowing		
MEDICAL SOCIAL WORK Expected Number of Visits: 1	❏ Review patient's financial status ❏ Make patient aware of care options ❏ Assess psychological needs	Instruct patient and caregiver in and establish home program on financial resources, self-help groups, and psychosocial needs	Improved understanding of funding sources and care options and reinforced therapeutic programing		

Source: Copyright © 1998, Cecil G. Betros, Jr.

Exhibit 8–5 Clinical Pathway Variance Report

Patient Name: _____ MR#: _____ Admission Date: _____ Initial POC: _____

Clinician: _____ ☐ RPT ☐ OTR ☐ SLP Agency: _____ Anticipated D/C date: _____

Primary Diagnosis: _____

Date	Therapist Initial	Variance Code	Patient Problem Affected	Action Taken/Comments

continues

Exhibit 8–5 continued

VARIANCE SYSTEMS AND CODES

1. Patient/Family	2. Practitioner	3. System External	4. System Internal
1.1 Refusal to participate in care	2.1 Practitioner error (explanation needed)	3.1 Home environment unsafe	4.1 Equipment breakdown
1.2 Nonproductive family dynamics	2.2 Error in discharge planning	3.2 Pt DC to hospital	4.2 Other
1.3 Conflicting appts other than MD		3.3 Pt DC to nursing home	
1.4 Unscheduled MD appts		3.4 Pt DC to inpatient rehab	
1.5 Exacerbation of patient dx		3.5 Pt DC to outpatient rehab	
1.6 Inability to progress activity R/T pain		3.6 Pt expired	
1.7 Unrelated sickness prevents participation in tx		3.7 Nonrenewal of MD orders	
1.8 Patient self-DC		3.8 Insurance benefits expired	
1.9 Pt out of service area for part of tx period		3.9 DC to another agency	
1.10 Pt expired		3.10 Pt moved out of service area	
1.11 Pt no longer homebound		3.11 Delay in insurance authorization for care	
1.12 Pt plateau in progress; max function achieved			
1.13 Pt reached goals earlier than expected			
1.14 Pt unavailable (explanation needed)			

Source: Copyright © 1998, Cecil G. Betros, Jr.

care can become continuous and standardized. When measuring quality, third-party payers, surveying organizations, and many managed care companies strongly focus on patient goals and the desired outcome of patient care. Pathways provide the formula necessary to govern utilization of professional services based on patient need. Speech-language pathologists, in conjunction with the agencies they service, should develop pathways that are specific for the patients they treat.

Home care reimbursement is moving toward providing payment for patient outcomes of care rather than patient visits. The pathway will enable speech-language pathologists to be included in the payment system and will provide critical information to the agency, which must link costs with actual care given. Because all providers of service will be competing within the managed care environment, the pathway will ensure a systematic, quality-driven system.

COMPETENCY ASSESSMENT

Competency assessment is absolutely essential for any organization. The current initiative in this area is for home health agencies to find employees or contractors qualified to meet the needs of their patients. Before an agency can assign staff to care for patients, it must be sure that the staff person assigned has the competency and skill level to care for that particular patient. A competency system is an ongoing process that begins with the job application and continues throughout the employee's entire tenure with the agency.

Changes in health care, advances in medical technology, and changes in health care delivery systems make it imperative that speech-language pathologists keep up-to-date with their competencies. Managed care has had a major impact on home health. Patients are being discharged from the hospital after just a few days. Patients who were formerly in intensive care units are now receiving home care. These complex care issues add to the need to ensure ongoing competency.

A critical assessment of competencies is the beginning point for any agency to determine which candidates are likely to succeed in home care. Excellent assessment skills and technical competencies are absolutely essential. Good common sense and an understanding of norms facilitate the transition to home care for clinicians from other settings or new graduates. Typically, an agency establishes the competencies that are necessary to care for its patients with significant input from the speech-language pathologist. In large group practices, a common practice is for the speech-language pathologist to submit speech-language pathology criteria for competence to the agency. In addition, the clinician and the agency establish systems to validate these competencies.

To test competence, an agency can use a pre- and postorientation examination in class and assess prospective clinicians' competence on basic cognitive and technical skills in the laboratory. Appendix 8–A is an example of a speech-language pathology competency assessment.

Competency assessment needs to be tailored to individual clinicians' practice patterns and the requirements of the agencies with which they deal. Before they are assigned to care for a patient alone, clinicians should demonstrate competency in the specific knowledge and skills that the patient will need.

Developing a competency system involves establishing standards, hiring appropriate speech-language pathologists, providing orientation, assessing ongoing competency, tracking data, and implementing systems to improve performance for individuals and groups. The challenge for the speech-language pathologist is to develop standards of care acceptable to the medical community and sanctioned by professional organizations and licensing boards. The most difficult task in developing these competencies is the fact that there are no definitive standards of care in the profession or standardized treatment methodologies. Unlike nurses, physical therapists, or occupational therapists, speech-language pathologists vary greatly in their ability to perform any given specific procedure, depending on the emphasis of their graduate-level education. In fact, this gap between education and practice has always existed. However, now that speech-language pathologists deal increasingly with patients in the acute phases of their illness and must meet the demand for improved health outcomes, educators should review their programs to determine how best to ensure the competency of clinicians entering the field and of those who currently practice.

REFERENCES

Bower, K. (1992). *Case management by nurses.* Washington, DC: American Nurses' Association.

Davis, (1994). Quality improvement. In M.D. Harris (Ed.), *Handbook of home health care administration.* Gaithersburg, MD: Aspen Publishers.

Gould, E., & Ruane, N. (1988). Components of a quality assurance program. In M. Harris, (Ed.), *Home health administration* (pp. 393–409). Owings Mills, MD: National Health Publishing.

Harris, M.D. (1994). *Handbook of home health care administration.* Gaithersburg, MD: Aspen Publishers.

Harris, M.D. (1997). *Handbook of home health care administration* (3rd ed.). Gaithersburg, MD: Aspen Publishers.

Joint Commission on Accreditation of Healthcare Organizations. (1993). *Quality improvement in home care.* Oakbrook, IL: Author.

Joint Commission on Accreditation of Healthcare Organizations. (1996). *1997–1998 Comprehensive accreditation manual for home care.* Oakbrook Terrace, IL: Author.

Prospective Payment Assessment Commission (ProPac). (1996). *Medicare and the American health care system: Report to Congress.* Washington, DC: Author.

Shaughnessy, P.W. (1991). *Shaping policy for long-term care: Learning from the effectiveness of hospital swing beds.* Ann Arbor, MI: Health Administration Press.

Shaughnessy, P.W., et al. (1994). Measuring and assuring the quality of home care. *Health Care Financing Review, 16,* 35–68.

Shaughnessy, P.W., & Crisler, K.S. (1995). *Outcome-based quality improvement.* Washington, DC: National Association for Home Care.

Shaughnessy, P.W., et al. (1995). Outcome-based quality improvement in home care. *Caring, 14,* 44–49.

Shaughnessy, P.W., et al. (1996). Home health care: Moving forward with continuous quality improvement. *Journal of Aging and Social Policy, 7,* 149–167.

Taber's cyclopedic medical dictionary. (1989). Philadelphia: F.A. Davis.

Zander, K. (1988). Nursing case management: Strategic management of cost and quality outcomes. *Journal of Nursing Administration, 18* (5), 23–30.

Zander, K. (1989). Managed care: Integrating QA in everyday practice. *Definition, 5,* 1–2.

Zander, K. (1993). Quantifying, managing and improving quality. Part IV: The retrospective use of variance. *New Definition, 8,* 1–3.

SUGGESTED READING

Bower, K. (1988). Managed care: Controlling costs, guaranteeing outcome. *Definition, 3* (3), 1–3.

Crisler, K.S., et al. (1994). *Objective review criteria for abstracting data for clinical record review of home health care* (Vol. 3). Denver, CO: University of Colorado Health Sciences Center, Center for Health Services Research.

Goodwin, D. (1992). Critical pathways in home healthcare. *Journal of Nursing Administration, 22* (2), 35–40.

McKenzie, C., et al. (1989). Care and cost: Nursing case management improves both. *Nursing Management, 20,* 30–34.

National Association for Home Care (NAHC). (1995). Medicare's OASIS: Standardized outcome and assessment information set for home health care. *NAHC Report* (Special Supplement No. 625, August 11). Washington, DC: Author.

Shaughnessy, P.W., et al. (1994). *Measuring outcomes of home health care* (Vol. 1). Denver, CO: Center for Health Policy Research.

Shaughnessy, P.W., et al. (1995). *Outcome based quality improvement: A manual for home care agencies on how to use outcomes.* Washington, DC: National Association of Home Care.

Clinical Competency Appraisal: Speech-Language Pathology

❏ **Orientation**   ❏ **Annual**   ❏ **Follow-Up**

Name:_____ **Date:** _____

Completed by: _____

Competency	Met	Not Met	Signature
Adult Assessment			
Manual Muscle Testing of the Oral-Facial Muscles			
Emergency Procedures: Syncopal Episode			
Ascertaining Subjective Information during an Initial Evaluation			
Geriatric Population			
Functional Communication Evaluation and Treatment			
Bedside Dysphagia Evaluation			

Competency: Adult Assessment (formal and informal testing)
Competency Statement: Demonstrates the ability to perform an adult assessment/differential diagnostic testing and is able to verbalize results in a concise summary.

Courtesy of Baptist Home Health Services, Inc., Birmingham, Alabama.

	Met	Not Met
1. Evaluation material is appropriate for diagnosis and current communication disorder.		
2. Uses infection control standards when appropriate.		
3. Is able to adjust testing material and criteria when patient is unable to respond to test items.		
4. Is able to correlate test data to function.		
5. Verbalizes diagnostic summary for patient/ caregiver in a concise and understandable manner.		

Competency Performed in:
❏ Clinical Setting
❏ Field Setting

❏ Passed
❏ Needs To Repeat

Date: _____

Employee: _____

Validated by: _____

COMMENTS:

Competency: Manual Muscle Testing of the Oral-Facial Muscles
Competency Statement: Demonstrates the ability to perform a hands-on
                                            manual muscle test of the oral-facial muscles and
                                            scores muscle movement correctly.

	Met	Not Met
1. Completes a cursory examination using a penlight.		
2. Uses gloves, mask, and sterile tongue blade when examining the oral structures.		
3. Uses correct hand placement for testing.		
4. Is able to manually test the oral-facial muscles, elicit muscle responses, and score the muscle movement correctly.		

Competency Performed in:
❑ Clinical Setting
❑ Field Setting

❑ Passed   Date: _____
❑ Needs To Repeat   Employee: _____
                                            Validated by: _____

COMMENTS:

Competency: Emergency Procedures: Syncopal Episode
Competency Statement: Demonstrates appropriate response to a syncopal episode.

Scenario:

You are treating a patient with aphasia/dysphagia in her home. The patient suddenly complains of weakness and becomes pale and sweaty. Next the patient begins to slump and pass out. Role play the situation and the steps that you would follow.

	Met	*Not Met*
1. Calls for help if available and makes patient stable in chair. If patient was ambulating, brings chair to patient or clears floor of possible hazards.		
2. Lowers patient into the chair and tilts chair backward or gently lowers patient to the floor.		
3. Assesses blood pressure and pulse of the patient; tries to keep the patient alert and aroused. Determines if the patient is diabetic.		
4. Transfers the patient to the bed or supine position and elevates the legs above the level of the heart.		
5. Calls the patient's primary nurse or 911 if necessary.		
6. If patient is diabetic, determines need to give orange juice.		
7. Follows instructions from nurse or other. Keeps patient comfortable.		

Competency Performed in:
❏ Clinical Setting
❏ Field Setting

❏ Passed
❏ Needs To Repeat

Date: _____
Employee: _____
Validated by: _____

COMMENTS:

Competency:	Ascertaining Subjective Information during an Initial Evaluation	
Competency Statement:	Demonstrates ability to ascertain pertinent subjective information during an initial evaluation.	

Case Study

You are to see a new client referred to you by a primary care physician. The referral gives a lengthy list of medical problems as well as an order that says "Evaluate and treat for general weakness and leg pain." The patient was initially seen by the physical therapist, who determined that the patient needs a speech-language evaluation because the patient has complained of difficulty in swallowing and discomfort when chewing foods.

What information is important to ascertain and why?

	Met	Not Met
Identifies specifics regarding:		
1. Patient's pain while chewing		
a. onset and possible cause		
b. location		
c. aggravating factors		
d. easing factors		
e. description of pain		
f. constant or intermittent		
g. sleep disturbance patterns		
h. functional limitations		
i. prior occurrences		
j. pain variance with food consistencies		
2. Prior treatment		
a. what was effective		
b. what was ineffective		
3. Medication taken		
4. Tests performed with patient's understanding of results		
5. Other significant medical history		
6. Occupation or prior level activity		
a. limitation of intake due to swallowing difficulties		
b. limitation of food textures		
7. Patient's stated goals		
a. realistic or not		
b. self-motivated or dependent		
c. psychological overlay present		

	Met	*Not Met*
8. Social history		
a. support systems		
b.other factors that affect outcome (family, finances, caregiving)		
c. how stress is handled		

Competency Performed in:
❑ Clinical Setting
❑ Field Setting

❑ Passed
❑ Needs To Repeat

Date: _____
Employee: _____
Validated by: _____

COMMENTS:

Competency: Geriatric Population
Competency Statement: Demonstrates an understanding of the unique issues
                                in the treatment of the geriatric population.

	Met	Not Met
1. Identifies factors that may contribute to cognitive problems in the geriatric population.		
2. Accepts geriatric patient's right to refuse treatment.		
3. Complies with geriatric patient's right to choose therapist, if feasible.		
4. Justifies recommendation for discharge of the geriatric patient on the basis of patient's and family's goals and wishes, cognitive abilities, social and financial support, and environmental considerations.		

Case Study

An 82-year-old white female was admitted to an agency with frequent falls. She was discharged from the hospital after falling in her home. Cause of the fall is unknown. She also presents with a T10 compression fracture and occasional dizziness. Past medical history: osteoporosis with severe thoracic kyphosis of the spine, high blood pressure. Social history: widowed for three months, no other family. Patient lives alone in a large two-story house with a bedroom and bathroom on the second floor. Financial: Medicare/Medicaid, lives on meager monthly Social Security check. Initial medical orders called for physical therapist (PT) and occupational therapist (OT) to instruct in donning Jewett brace and activities of daily life (ADLs), gait training to return to premorbid status. During the first physical therapy visit, the patient refused to finish the therapy session, stating that the male therapist who came to see her reminds her of her deceased husband. She would prefer a female therapist. After three weeks of physical and occupational therapy (at three times per week), the patient still cannot remember how to don her brace or how to "log-roll" for back protection; she is having difficulty in doing sequencing activities for ADLs and instrumental ADLs; her ambulation is limited to 25 feet with a rolling walker, when she remembers to use it, and minimal assistance of one, secondary to pain; she is unable to ascend stairs. The PT and OT both referred the patient to speech therapy for evaluation.

Questions

1. What factors may have contributed to the patient's falls in terms of communication disorders?
2. How do you handle her refusal to work with a male therapist?

3. How can the speech therapist establish a plan so that the PT and OT can meet the initial request by the physician?
4. What kind of planning do you recommend for the patient regarding continuation/discontinuation of therapy services? What discharge planning do you recommend? How do you justify your recommendations?

❏ Passed
❏ Needs To Repeat

Date: _____

Employee: _____

Validated by: _____

COMMENTS:

Competency: Functional Communication Evaluation and Treatment

Competency Statement: Demonstrates the ability to assess functional communication skills and develops a treatment plan geared to functional outcomes.

	Met	*Not Met*
1. Explains purpose of evaluation in terms of formal testing and relates the test data to functional communication.		
2. Assesses prior level of functional communication and home situation.		
3. Administers both formal and informal tests.		
4. Assesses current abilities to communicate basic wants and medical needs.		
5. Observes communication with family or caregiver.		
6. Establishes functional communication goals with patient and caregiver.		

Competency Performed in:
❑ Clinical Setting
❑ Field Setting

❑ Passed
❑ Needs To Repeat

Date: _____
Employee: _____
Validated by: _____

COMMENTS:

Competency: Bedside Dysphagia Evaluation
Competency Statement: Demonstrates appropriate and safe techniques when conducting a bedside dysphagia evaluation.

	Met	Not Met
1. Identifies factors that are important to the patient's swallowing.		
a. Prior MBS		
b. Consistencies that present problems to the patient		
c. Prior history of swallowing difficulties		
d. Patient's description of problem		
2. Is able to assess baseline vital signs (temperature, pulse, respiration, blood pressure).		
3. Uses standard infection control measures during evaluation.		
4. Evaluates patient at bedside using accepted standards of practice in regard to administration of oral intake.		
5. Assesses neuromuscular control of the oral-facial muscles using the Manual Muscle Testing Method.		
6. Discusses the dysphagia program with the patient or caregiver with special reference to		
a. patient safety while swallowing		
b. compensatory strategies, if appropriate		
c. referral for MBS if indicated		
d. diet consistency		
e. home exercise program		
f. ensuring that family and/or caregiver is trained in choking precautions		
7. Observes patient eating a typical consistency used in his or her everyday diet.		
8. Makes appropriate referral to other disciplines as indicated.		

Competency Performed in:
❑ Clinical Setting
❑ Field Setting

❑ Passed
❑ Needs To Repeat

Date: _____
Employee: _____
Validated by: _____

PART IV

The Future

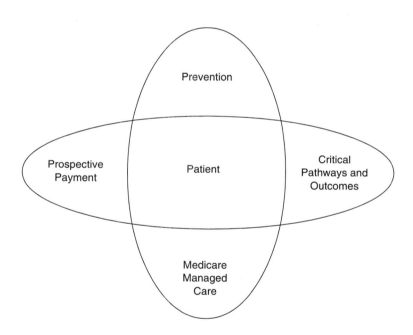

Implications of the Interim Payment System on the Practice of Speech-Language Pathology in Home Health

BACKGROUND

The Balanced Budget Act (BBA) of 1997 was enacted in August 1997, and the interim payment system (IPS) became effective October 1, 1997. The IPS was designed to reduce projected expenditures for Medicare home health care services for fiscal years 1998 and 1999 (Prospective Payment Assessment Commission, 1996). The IPS reduces per visit cost limits on the average of 21 percent, and the new per beneficiary limit will result in a reduction in the average spending per Medicare patient (Bishop & Skwara, 1993). Given that the IPS is untested, the full impact on Medicare beneficiaries and home care providers is unclear. The IPS is expected to slow the growth of Medicare home health care expenditures and possibly move toward a somewhat more uniform benefit. However, the IPS raises some concerns about the impact on beneficiaries, home health care providers, and practicing clinicians, including questions about access to home health care services, quality of care, and continued viability of home health agencies.

In response to the IPS, most home health agencies have had to reduce costs per visit and costs per patient. The actions taken may either directly or indirectly affect Medicare home health care users. Because 78 percent of an agency's costs are labor related, the reductions in the payment ceilings could mean that agencies may not be able to increase employee wages and fringe benefits to keep pace with cost-of-living increases. In addition, contracting therapists will likely have a reduction in their per visit rate equal to that of agency reductions. Such reductions may make home health care agencies less attractive to potential employees and to contracting therapists and therapy groups.

The new per beneficiary limit also creates pressure to reduce the amount of services provided, which could have a more direct impact on home health patients and contract speech-language pathologists. The per beneficiary limit is applied in the aggregate, so it does not matter if any particular beneficiary has costs higher than the limit, as long as on average the agency's cost is below the limit. However, to remain below the limit, agencies will need to focus on reducing per patient costs and maintaining a low cost mix of patients. For the speech-language pathologist, this will mean an obvious reduction in the amount of time (length of stay) and the amount of visits per patient. Since most of the patients seen in home health care by speech-language pathologists have neurological problems that require extensive intervention, limiting the visits per patient episode would result in an overall cost reduction.

With this concept in mind, speech-language pathologists need to to adopt one or more of several strategies:

- Where medically appropriate, home health care agencies could reduce the number of visits provided to patients. Agencies will likely target high-use patients for reductions. Speech-language pathologists must be able to treat patients effectively and efficiently. They may use home exercises and train caregivers and family to carry out daily, repetitive exercises. They might use assistants to reduce the costs.
- Home health care agencies could reduce the average number of visits and cost per patient without rationing care by increasing the number of persons served (volume), focusing on individuals with lower than average numbers of visits (such as orthopaedic patients). However, any additional patients would still be required to meet the Medicare coverage guidelines, so the pool of potential new home health users may be limited. The key here is volume. Speech-language pathologists must market their services and assist agencies in identifying patients in order to increase the volume, reduce the length of stay, and maintain the same reimbursement structure.
- Home health care agencies could reduce their average number of visits and cost per patient by serving fewer high-use/high-cost patients (i.e., involved stroke patients). As a result, speech-language pathologists could see a reduction in the actual number of patients with long-term neurological implications who are referred for services.
- Home health care agencies could use several substitution strategies to reduce the average cost per beneficiary. These strategies include reducing more expensive visits in favor of lower cost visits where appropriate (e.g., substituting licensed practical nurses for registered nurses and therapy assistants for therapists) and combining services within one visit to the extent possible (multiskilling). These strategies have to be carefully implemented in appropriate situations, or they could negatively affect patient outcomes. Speech-language pathologists who are not familiar with routine medical assessment

need to learn how to assess basic vital signs, skin integrity, and so forth, since they likely will be asked to participate in a multiskilling approach to patient care.

- Home health care agencies could establish protocols and frequent status reviews in an effort to limit the possibility of providing an excessive number of visits. Speech-language pathologists must become familiar with critical pathways and outcome management procedures in order to survive. The clinician should use actual clinical data in determining outcomes. In addition, the clinician must show how treatment has affected the patient's health status or independence.

Those patients with long stays and/or high use are particularly likely to receive fewer visits or may have difficulty accessing care. In 1994, Medicare beneficiaries who received 200 or more visits were more likely to have medically complex needs, use extensive inpatient hospital care, and require multiple home health care episodes (Kenney, 1991). They were also more likely to have severe functional impairments. On the basis of the available data, it is not possible to determine the amount of service reduction that can be accomplished without negative outcomes. Patients with this profile who are unable to access home health services are likely to use other services, such as nursing home or hospital care, or possibly seek Medicaid-covered home care. Previously, high-use patients who disagreed with noncoverage determinations had the protection of medical review processes and appeals. Under the IPS, beneficiaries who potentially could use a high level of service and cannot access home health services do not have an appeals process available to secure services from an agency.

Because of increases in the number of visits per user since 1993/1994 (the base year for the per beneficiary limits), nearly all home health agencies will likely need to adopt at least one of the preceding strategies. The changes in the payment structure could have an effect on the type of patients agencies are financially able to serve and, as a result, may also disrupt the established patterns of referrals. Although the provisions of this system could encourage agencies and/or the government to develop and implement protocols and guidelines that have the potential to reduce services and cost without adversely affecting patients, for many agencies this will take time and require enhanced data on patient characteristics, utilization, and outcomes.

THE MEDICARE HOME HEALTH BENEFIT

Medicare covers the skilled services of nursing care, physical therapy, occupational therapy, speech-language pathology services, and medical social services under the home health benefit. If a beneficiary receives skilled home health services from a nurse or therapist, he or she may also receive care from a home health aide for services such as assistance with bathing. Medicare requires services to be authorized by physician orders for individuals under the care of a physician who are homebound and need intermittent skilled nursing, physical therapy, or speech-pathology services. Nursing and home health aide services must be furnished on a part-time (generally less than eight hours a day) or an intermittent basis (generally less than seven days a week). Medicare beneficiaries are not required to have a hospital stay prior to receiving home health care, and there is no copayment or deductible associated with the benefit.

Medicare currently reimburses home health agencies on a cost basis, subject to limits. Prior to October 1, 1997, the limit was 112 percent of the average of the labor-related and nonlabor unit costs of free-standing home health agencies for each of the covered disciplines (nursing, physical therapy, occupational therapy, speech-language pathology services, medical social services, and home health aide services). The limit is applied in the aggregate. This means that an agency's total allowable costs for all visits must be equal to or less than the sum of the cost limits by discipline multiplied by the number of visits the agency provided for each discipline.

Medicare home health services became a target for reductions as a result of the growth in expenditures. Medicare home health expenditures grew rapidly over the past several years after relatively slow growth during most of the 1980s. Recently, however, the rate of growth dropped from between 20 and 50 percent to 5 percent from 1996 to 1997. The majority of the growth in expenditures resulted from increases in the number of visits per home health user and the number of home health users per 1,000 Medicare beneficiaries. In response to the growth in use per beneficiary, the new per beneficiary limit of the IPS places limits on the overall average costs per patient (Kenney, 1991).

BALANCED BUDGET ACT OF 1997

The BBA provides for reductions in existing cost limits and changes in reimbursement with the establishment of a new per beneficiary cost limit, followed by a prospective payment system (PPS). On the basis of its 1997 baseline, the Congressional Budget Office (CBO) estimated that these changes would save $16.1 billion through 2002.

Interim Payment System

The IPS for Medicare home health services reduces the per visit cost limits and institutes a per beneficiary annual limit. Initially two changes are made to the per visit cost limits:

1. Elimination of market basket update for the period of the freeze on cost limits effective 1994 to 1996. The market basket update granted in 1996 following the two-year freeze on the cost limits was eliminated. This means that changes in costs between July 1994 and July 1996 would not be accounted for in the cost limits.
2. Cost limits based on 105 percent of the median cost per visit of free-standing agencies rather than the previous 112 percent of the mean.

The per beneficiary limit will be calculated based on 75 percent of the agency's reasonable cost per beneficiary and on 25 percent of the census division average reasonable cost per beneficiary. These calculations will be made using 98 percent of reasonable costs for cost reporting periods ending in federal fiscal year 1994, including nonroutine medical supplies, and updated by the home health market basket index, excluding the freeze period. Many agencies use the calendar year for their fiscal year, which will result in a per beneficiary limit based on 1993 information. Those providers without a base year cost report will be assigned the median of these limits. The per beneficiary limit will be applied in the aggregate, so it does not matter if any particular beneficiary has costs higher than the limit, as long as on average the agency's cost is below the limit.

Under the IPS, home health agencies will be paid the lowest of the following (Kenney, 1991):

- the actual allowable costs of providing services
- the aggregated reduced per visit cost limits
- an aggregated per beneficiary annual limit

These provisions are in effect for cost reporting periods beginning between October 1997 and September 1999.

Prospective Payment System

The BBA of 1997 calls for a full PPS for cost reporting periods beginning in October 1999. The Health Care Financing Administration (HCFA) has not yet developed any of the details of the PPS, only that payments will be based on the most current audited cost reports. The PPS will most likely be a per episode payment adjusted for case mix. The BBA calls for a 15 percent reduction in home health limits beginning October 1, 1999, whether or not a PPS has been implemented.

IMPACT OF KEY PROVISIONS ON BENEFICIARIES

Although the full impact of the payment changes on beneficiaries is unknown, certain aspects of the IPS raise concerns about access to care, shifting of care to less appropriate settings, lack of alternative financing sources, increases in beneficiary out-of-pocket payments, and reduced quality of care. Only careful monitoring of the IPS will reveal whether any necessary reductions to stay below the limits can be accomplished without negative consequences for beneficiaries.

In response to the IPS, home health agencies will need to reduce cost per visit and cost per patient. The actions taken may either directly or indirectly affect Medicare home health users.

Potentially Reduced Availability of Home Care for High-Intensity Cases

To the extent a case will likely exceed the per beneficiary annual limit, home health agencies may have an incentive to reduce the level of care provided to these individuals, either by shifting the mix of care to a lower cost skill mix or by reducing the number of visits provided. Those with long stays or high use would be most likely to receive fewer visits. In addition, some high-cost patients may be unable to access home health services if agencies are fearful of the financial impact of admitting them for services.

Previous research on use of the home health benefit indicates that the sicker and more frail beneficiaries are likely to be the most vulnerable to reductions. In 1994, 10 percent of Medicare home health recipients received 200 or more visits and accounted for 43 percent of total Medicare home health expenditures (Leon, Neuman, & Paranet, 1997). These types of patients may have difficulty accessing services or experience reductions in service. Medicare beneficiaries who received 200 or more visits were more likely to have medically complex needs, use extensive inpatient hospital care, and require multiple home health care episodes. They were also more likely to have severe functional impairments. Consistent with the profile of recipients with chronic needs, these high-use patients received considerably more home health aide visits than the average home health beneficiary—206 versus 36 visits, on average. They also used more skilled nursing services—101 versus 30 visits. Systematic analyses of data concerning patient characteristics, outcomes, and utilization are needed to determine whether reductions in service occur and, if so, the impact of the reductions.

The Medicare program provides a mechanism for beneficiaries receiving home health services to appeal a denial of services through medical review processes and appeals. However, if the IPS leads to denial of admission for high-use patients, then those patients have no appeals process available to secure services from an agency. Individuals who believe they have been denied admission but meet coverage criteria can file a complaint with Medicare. However, while the Medicare program could terminate an agency if it determines the agency wrongfully discriminated against a patient, the agency cannot be compelled to provide services. Therefore, under current regulations, there is no appeal process that will guarantee access to home health services.

Shifting of Care to Potentially Less Appropriate Settings

If access to care is reduced, hospital and nursing home admissions could increase, particularly for those without family or other community supports. Patients without informal caregivers receive more Medicare home health visits than those with informal caregivers (Williams, 1994). If Medicare home health becomes less available, these individuals may have to seek care elsewhere. Patients in the East South Central region (Alabama, Kentucky, Mississippi, and Texas) may be more likely to enter nursing homes because of the lack of alternative community-based services in this region (Schore, 1994).

Possible Lack of Alternative Financing Sources for Care

Even though over one-third of home health recipients with 200 or more visits have Medicaid coverage, reductions in expected Medicaid expenditures may limit access to Medicaid home and community-based care and also make nursing home care a less viable alternative option, potentially increasing unmet need. On the other hand, as states search for ways to reduce total Medicaid expenditures by shifting care to lower cost settings, Medicaid coverage for home and community-based care may increase.

Possible Increases in Beneficiary Out-of-Pocket Payments

As a result of limited alternative sources of third-party payments for home care, if beneficiaries experience reductions in Medicare coverage that they need to function independently in their home, they will likely have to pay for that care from their own resources or they could experience unmet need. Increasing the out-of-pocket expenditure for home care will be limited by both the patient's ability to pay and the willingness of other family members to provide assistance. Having to finance care from personal resources could be particularly problematic for those with high numbers of home health visits, the beneficiaries most likely to be affected, because 80 percent of these individuals have annual income less than $15,000 (Leon et al., 1997).

More Uniform Benefits

Basing one-quarter of the per beneficiary limit on the average for the census division serves as an incentive to agencies to provide a level of care more similar to the census division average. This could partially move the Medicare home health benefit toward a more uniform benefit, at least within a census division. This provision would not be expected to reduce the variation in home health expenditures per beneficiary among the census divisions. It also only partially addresses the variation within a census division. Basing the per beneficiary limit on 75 percent of agency-specific per beneficiary costs can still result in wide variations in the limits applied to agencies within the same market.

IMPACT OF KEY PROVISIONS ON HOME HEALTH AGENCIES

The pressures for home health agencies under the IPS will be to hold down costs per visit and cost per patient. Cost per patient is influenced by both cost per visit and number of visits provided. In response, agencies may try to increase the proportion of low-end users with fewer visits and to restrain the overall average number of visits to approximately 1993/1994 levels so that an agency's aggregate cost is below the lower of the two limits. The primary binding constraint on reimbursement for most home health agencies will be the new per beneficiary limit, which will likely result in fewer visits per home health user on average than in recent years.

Reduce Per Visit Costs

The reduction of the per visit limits from 112 percent of the mean cost per visit to 105 percent of the median cost per visit requires agencies to seriously examine their cost structures. The published new per visit cost limits and the resulting lower budget neutrality adjustment are on average 21 percent lower than what the limits would have been without the IPS. J. Jensen, a Congressional Budget Office analyst for Medicare home health, estimates that the proportion of home health agencies exceeding the per visit cost limits will increase from approximately 30 percent prior to the change to nearly two-thirds following the reduction (personal communication, February 4, 1998). Hospital-based agencies, particularly those in urban areas, are the most likely to exceed the cost limits. The per beneficiary limit increases the likelihood that an agency will have costs that exceed its per visit limit because as agencies decrease the volume of visits, the unit cost per visit will likely increase. If agencies are unable to make necessary cost reductions, they will experience financial losses and potential closure.

Since almost 78 percent of visit costs are labor related, the reductions in the payment ceilings could mean that some agencies may not be able to increase employee wages and fringe benefits to keep pace with cost-of-living increases or retain higher cost personnel. Such action may make these agencies less attractive to potential employees.

As agencies prepare for the PPS, they will also need to consider updating their reporting and tracking mechanisms by possibly computerizing them at a time when they may need to reduce overhead expenditures. These cost reductions may also make it more difficult for agencies to invest in new technology, upgrade computer systems, and so forth.

Restrain the Overall Average Number of Visits to 1993/1994 Levels

The per beneficiary cost limit specifies a blend based 75 percent on agency-specific data and 25 percent on the census division average. The use of the agency-specific portion was intended to serve as a crude adjustment for the historical case mix of an agency. The use of the census division portion, rather than a national average, acknowledges regional variation in home health service use. While agency case mix would not be expected to change significantly from year to year, the use of four- to five-year-old data to adjust for case mix fails to reflect changes in the mix of patients since the base year. The IPS has no specific mechanism to adjust for agency changes in the mix of patients.

In order to remain below the per beneficiary limit, agencies will need to focus on maintaining a low cost mix of patients. The dramatic growth in the average number of visits per client since 1993/1994 could make this difficult. The average number of visits per patient increased 34 percent from calendar year 1993 to calendar year 1996 (from 59 to 79 visits per patient) and 15 percent from calendar year 1994 to calendar year 1996 (Bishop & Skwara, 1993). Medicare coverage guidelines have not changed, with the exception of the removal of venipuncture as a qualifying skilled service. Agencies could adopt one or more of several strategies.

- Where medically appropriate, home health agencies could reduce the number of visits provided to patients.
- Home health agencies could reduce the average number of visits per user without rationing care by increasing the number of persons served (volume), focusing on individuals with lower than average numbers of visits. This could be challenging because the percentage of Medicare beneficiaries using home health benefits increased from just under 6 percent to over 9 percent from 1990 to 1995 (Kenney & Moon, 1997); therefore, the pool of potential new beneficiaries could be tapped out. Medicare payment reductions to hospitals included in the BBA might result in more hospital discharges referred for home health care. However, hospitals that transfer patients to home care or other subacute services face the possibility of revenue reductions under a new transfer provision in the BBA that authorizes reductions in the diagnosis-

related group (DRG) rate for hospitals that make transfers to subacute care.

- Home health agencies could use several substitution strategies to reduce the average expenditure per beneficiary.
- Home health agencies could establish care protocols and frequent status reviews in an effort to limit the possibility of providing an excessive number of visits.

Because of increases in the number of visits per user since 1993/1994, nearly all home health agencies will likely need to adopt at least one of these strategies. To the extent that agencies provide fewer visits, staff may have to be laid off.

Home health agencies most affected by the new per beneficiary limit include (1) those that have had an increase in severity in their case mix since 1994, requiring either more visits or a higher proportion of nursing or therapy visits; (2) small agencies serving a large number of high-use patients that cannot balance their use with increases in patients with lesser use; (3) rural agencies where alternative sources of care are less likely to be available; (4) agencies that have added services since 1994 that will not be included in the per beneficiary limit calculation; and (5) agencies that are the result of mergers or acquisitions where the surviving provider number's historical experience reflects lower per beneficiary limits than the combined mix of patients and services (Kenney & Moon, 1997).

Other Expected Effects on Operations

The payment changes would be expected to have the following effects on other aspects of home health agency operations:

- *Potential changes to the nature of competition within a market*—The recent changes in the payment structure will have an effect on agency incentives for the type of patients agencies would prefer to serve and, as a result, will disrupt the established patterns of referrals. Many home health patients are referred to an agency by hospital discharge planners. Currently, each agency in a market will try to establish a particular niche in the market (e.g., high-tech care or care requiring home health aides), and discharge planners and physicians will generally base referral patterns on established strengths of agencies. It will take time for the agencies, physicians, and hospital discharge planners to reconfigure referral patterns in response to the new system. In addition, the per beneficiary limits may vary substantially within the same market. This may encourage agencies with higher per beneficiary limits to market their services on the basis of an ability to provide more services than competitors provide. This may put the agency with a low cost per patient in the base year at a competitive disadvantage.

- *New data requirements*—Effective for cost reporting periods beginning on or after October 1, 1997, the BBA requires home health agencies to submit additional information that the Secretary of the Department of Health and Human Services considers necessary for the development of a reliable case-mix system. Likely data elements include impairment in activities of daily living (ADLs), specific diagnoses, and other Outcome and Assessment Information Set (OASIS) data items.
- *Development of more responsive data systems*—For agencies to effectively manage care under the new payment system, they will need systems to track care provided to beneficiaries more closely. Agencies will also have a more immediate need for information in order to monitor the financial implications of the type and level of care provided. Agencies that have incorporated OASIS data collection into their system will be ahead of the game.
- *Possible development of systematic guidelines for care*—The IPS encourages agencies to provide less care and/or substitute lesser skilled, lower cost providers. These lower cost providers, generally home health aides, require more monitoring and supervision. Agencies may turn to care guidelines to assist them in this process. Agencies will also consider methods to manage utilization, such as case management, utilization review, and standardized protocols for care.

While each of these operational changes may result in increased efficiencies, they may also impose costs on agencies. An example is that new data requirements may require an agency to incur costs related to modifying its information systems. Given the reductions in the cost limits, agencies may not be able to defray these costs, and thus may not have the resources to adapt.

Approximately two-thirds of agencies have fiscal years beginning October through January and had four months' or less notice of the reimbursement changes. Agencies that cannot adapt rapidly to these changes will face financial losses and/or closure. These closures could reduce access to home health services in particular areas. This is of particular concern in rural areas where access to home health services is less plentiful.

Transition to the Prospective Payment System

The incentives for home health agencies under a PPS will likely be somewhat similar to those under the IPS. However, rather than just recovering their costs, agencies will have the potential to earn profit from Medicare as hospitals do under the PPS for hospitals. A per episode PPS would require agencies to monitor costs of care and the number of visits provided to beneficiaries, similar to the per visit and per beneficiary limits. One major difference under the PPS will be a method to adjust payments to account for an agency's level of severity of clients served. Instituting a case-mix adjustment should alleviate the pressures to reduce visits for patients who require more complex care or those who are chronically ill. The extent of the relief depends on the degree to which the case-mix adjuster reflects variations in care delivery, the nature of the definition of an episode, and the outlier payment policy under the PPS.

QUALITY OF CARE

The responses of home health agencies to the new Medicare reimbursement system could have implications for quality of care. The lack of any systematic quality assurance mechanisms in the IPS could be problematic. Even if the IPS included new quality assurance mechanisms, the lack of accepted standards for the quantity and recommended providers of home health services hinders efforts to address the appropriateness of potential service reductions. Of particular concern is the potential for curtailed episodes, provider substitution, increased staff turnover, and disrupted referral patterns.

Where medically appropriate, home health agencies could reduce the number of visits provided to patients. As indicated earlier, agencies would likely target high-use patients for reductions. If an agency's visits per patient experience was similar to the national rate of growth, and the agency did not serve any additional low-use patients and was not able to reduce costs in other ways, the per beneficiary limit could require reducing visits by 15 percent to 30 percent. Evidence suggests that patients with curtailed episodes may have poorer outcomes. Medicare patients with managed care were found to have fewer visits, shorter home health stays, and poorer outcomes than those of fee-for-service patients (Shaughnessy, Schlenker, & Hittle, 1994).

Home health agencies could also use several substitution strategies to reduce the average expenditure per beneficiary. These strategies include reducing more expensive visits in favor of lower cost visits where appropriate (e.g., substituting licensed practical nurses for registered nurses and therapy assistants for therapists); combining services within one visit to the extent possible; and using telephone follow-up. Agencies will need to take care when using these strategies so that quality is not adversely affected.

In addition, reduced per visit cost limits may cause some agencies to reduce agency employees' pay and/or fringe benefits. This, in turn, may make these agencies less attractive to potential employees with appropriate skills for home health care and further increase turnover. Less experienced providers with high turnover rates could affect both the continuity and quality of care.

Finally, disruptions in referral patterns could also impact quality of care. These may result as agencies seek to identify lower cost patient referral sources. Disruptions in discharge plan implementation that includes planned home health care services are a significant predictor of negative outcomes (e.g., rehospitalization and unmet needs) (Proctor, Morrow-Howell, & Kaplan, in press).

To encourage the maintenance of quality, home health agencies could establish care protocols and frequent status reviews in an effort to limit the possibility of providing excessive numbers of visits. However, for those agencies that have not already adopted the data systems and processes for monitoring patient care, it will take enhanced data on patient characteristics, utilization, and outcomes to develop these.

BUDGETARY IMPACT ESTIMATES

On the basis of its 1997 baseline, the CBO estimated that the IPS would reduce Medicare home health payments $3.1 billion in fiscal years 1998 and 1999. The PPS was expected to reduce payments an additional $13.0 billion over the baseline during the 2000 to 2002 period. In January 1998, the CBO revised its baseline projections to incorporate the most recently available data. The growth rate for 1996 to 1997 sharply decelerated, changing from a projected 13 percent to only 4.8 percent. As a result of this modest increase in Medicare home health payments between 1996 and 1997, the CBO lowered its baseline spending projections, resulting in expected total expenditures for Medicare home health of $37.5 billion rather than $41.2 billion between 1998 and 1999 (Table 9–1). The CBO's most recent budget projections indicate that the required 15 percent reduction in limits in fiscal year 2000 are expected to result in a reduction in Medicare home health spending.

In developing its projections of the impact of any proposal, the CBO develops estimates of the impact based on the legislative language and accounts for any expected changes in provider behavior that may offset the impact of the provisions. Under the IPS, the CBO analyst assumed that the effect of the new per beneficiary payment limit would produce only about one-third as much of a reduction as might be expected if utilization (the percentage of beneficiaries using home health) and intensity (the number of visits per beneficiary using home health) remained the same as under the baseline (J. Jensen, CBO analyst, telephone conversation, February 4, 1998). This means that $9.3 billion in reductions, assuming no behavioral response under the IPS, are scored as $3.1 billion in savings. The offset of $6.2 billion is used to account for home health agencies' recruiting additional

Table 9–1 CBO Estimates (in Billions of Dollars) of the Impact of Home Health Payment Changes

	1997	1998	1999	2000	2001	2002	1998–2002
1997 Baseline	$19.0	$21.1	$23.2	$25.3	$27.5	$29.9	$127.0
Policy change		–$1.1	–$2.0	–$4.1	–$4.2	–$4.7	–$16.1
New Home Health	$19.0	$20.0	$21.2	$21.2	$23.3	$25.2	$110.9
1998 Baseline	$17.5	$18.2	$19.3	$19.0	$21.4	$23.1	$101.0

Source: Congressional Budget Office, *Economic and Budget Outlook: Fiscal Years 1998–2007,* January 1997, a Memorandum on the impact of the Balanced Budget Act of 1997 dated August 12, 1997, and *Economic and Budget Outlook: Fiscal Years 1999–2008,* January 1998.

patients under the IPS. In 1999, the $4.0 billion offset translates into approximately one million additional users. This would be in addition to the HCFA projections of 4.3 million home health users in 1999 and implies an increase in use of the Medicare home health benefit from approximately 11 percent to 14 percent among Medicare fee-for-service beneficiaries.

The CBO analyst cited the lack of a mechanism to control the volume of patients served under the IPS as the rationale for assuming a two-thirds behavioral offset. The provisions of the BBA fail to encourage changes in the delivery of fee-for-service care so that services are provided in the most appropriate setting or that coordination systematically occurs across settings. In particular, the BBA's increased pressure on hospitals could increase referrals to home health agencies or to skilled nursing facilities, followed by referral to home health agencies upon discharge from a skilled nursing facility.

The CBO's offset assumption would be consistent with a rather large increase in hospital referrals to home health agencies. Approximately 20 percent of Medicare beneficiaries are admitted to a hospital each year. Eleven percent of those admitted to a hospital use the Medicare skilled nursing facility benefit, and nearly 14 percent use the Medicare home health benefit (Prospective Payment Assessment Commission, 1996). If the one million additional users all entered home health through a hospital discharge, this implies approximately 30 percent of Medicare fee-for-service beneficiaries using hospitals would also use home health. These new patients would likely use few home health visits and would lower an agency's average payments per beneficiary, making it easier to keep costs below the per beneficiary limit. However, these new patients would have to meet the Medicare home health coverage guidelines, and hospitals may be more reluctant to refer Medicare patients to subacute care since the transfer provision became effective in October 1998.

Although not explicitly accounted for in the CBO projections, the reductions in Medicare home health payments may result in an increase in Medicaid payments. Over one-third of home health users with 200 or more visits have Medicaid coverage (Leon et al., 1997). These individuals may be able to replace potential reductions in Medicare home health visits with Medicaid home health or home and community-based care. In many states, however, home and community-based waiver programs have a limited number of slots available and long waiting lists. This is particularly true in states with a high average number of Medicare home health visits. A subset of these states have actively exploited Medicare coverage for their dual eligibles in an effort to reduce Medicaid expenditures. If these patients do not receive adequate services to maintain them at home, they may need nursing home placement at the expense of state Medicaid programs. Therefore, the impact depends upon availability of home and community-based services and whether reduced home care services increase nursing home placements.

ADMINISTRATIVE ISSUES

The HCFA will have two major challenges related to the Medicare home health provisions included in the BBA. The first is calculating the per beneficiary limits and the second is developing a PPS within the time frame specified in the act.

Per Beneficiary Limits

Calculating the per beneficiary limit of the IPS requires information about the number of unduplicated Medicare beneficiaries served by a home health agency during agency fiscal years ending during federal fiscal year 1994 (October 1, 1993, to September 30, 1994). Although Medicare home health cost reports request a census count from agencies, many agencies appear to have reported admissions/discharges or left the field blank because this information was not used for reimbursement in previous years. Therefore, the only centralized approach to estimating the number of unduplicated Medicare beneficiaries served by individual home health agencies is to aggregate home health use at the beneficiary level for each home health agency during its relevant fiscal year. This requires the use of claims data for each home health agency for the period covered by the agency's fiscal year ending between October 1, 1993, and September 30, 1994. Making these calculations requires combining information from several databases across at least two years. In the interim, agencies will have completed up to six months of the cost reporting period without knowing the applicable per beneficiary limit. This may result in agencies' incurring costs for which they may not be reimbursed or taking the defensive strategy of avoiding admissions of and reducing services to high-cost patients when possible.

The consequences of not having an accurate per beneficiary limit could be problematic for home health agencies. If an agency reported admissions on its cost report, rather than unduplicated beneficiaries, this would reduce the agency-specific portion of its per beneficiary limit, causing further constraints on its cost limits. If an agency did not report a census count on its 1993/1994 cost report, or was founded after the applicable period, the HCFA must use a proxy. HCFA staff indicated they likely will use the national median per beneficiary limit (CBO, 1997). This could further restrict the cost limits for agencies in areas with higher than the median cost per patient and place little incentive to control use upon agencies in areas with lower than the median cost per patient. Also, given the skewed distribution of average reimbursement per beneficiary, the use of the median implies that the level will be lower than if the mean were to be used.

Transition to the Prospective Payment System

The BBA calls on the HCFA to develop and implement a home health PPS in approximately two years. The HCFA's episode-based PPS demonstration is not scheduled to be completed and evaluated until after the date the new PPS is to be implemented. This could make it difficult to test the necessary components of a PPS, including the impact of the case-mix groupings and the episode definition. Also, the project to develop the key component of a PPS, the case-mix adjuster, just began collecting data late in 1997, with the initial recommendations due January 1999.

A particular challenge for the HCFA will be developing a case-mix adjuster that reflects the cost of providing services to various types of patients. The current Medicare Home Health Prospective Payment Demonstration has 18 case-mix groupings designed to provide a comparison of the types of cases handled within an agency from year to year to adjust the agency-specific episode-based prospective payment rate. It was not designed to differentiate the intensity of cases for payment among agencies. Patient diagnoses account for only a small proportion of the variance in home health utilization (Goldberg & Schmitz, 1994). The PPS demonstration case-mix groupings account for less than 10 percent of the variation in utilization. In contrast, other payment systems that attempt to account for differences in resource use account for a much greater portion of the variation. The DRG system, when applied to all patients in acute care hospitals, explains about 30 percent of the variation in resource use (Cretin & Worthman, 1986; Schneider, Fries, Foley, Desmond, & Gormley, 1988). The pilot resource utilization groups (RUG) system, developed for nursing home payment in New York State, explained 37.8 percent of the resource variation (Fries & Cooney, 1985; Schneider et al., 1988), and further refinements have increased the proportion. Although not directly comparable, these provide a rough guide to the amount of variability typically explained by a case-mix system.

Another challenge for the HCFA will be revamping the medical review process for home health, particularly in light of potential accusations of patient dumping under prospective payment. Medical reviews have historically focused on medical necessity and will now be required to ensure appropriate service. It will be necessary to overhaul the current medical review system in a short period of time and possibly increase the number of reviews to meet the goal of appropriate service. Increasing the number of reviews would increase paperwork that must be requested. Protocols for medical review to satisfy the requirement to ensure appropriate service will need to be developed. This may have the advantage of speeding the development of new guidelines for care.

If the HCFA is unable to meet the October 1, 1999, deadline for implementing a home health PPS, it may be wise to consider a plan for evaluating the effect of the IPS on an ongoing basis. Areas for evaluation could include

- changes in the percentage of fee-for-service Medicare beneficiaries served, to monitor the extent to which agencies adapt to the new payment system by increasing the volume of patients they serve
- the characteristics of home health patients admitted under the IPS, to determine if the high-use/high-cost patients continue to have access to Medicare home health services, if there is a reduction in services provided, and if the IPS has an impact on patient outcomes or the use of other services
- the impact on the number, location, and type of Medicare-certified home health agencies
- potential methods to case-mix adjust the per beneficiary limit

Assessing these areas would provide the HCFA with information that could be used to modify payment to reduce unintended consequences and optimize patient care.

CONCLUSION

The IPS will have differential impacts on agencies and beneficiaries. Home health agencies that have had large increases in cost per beneficiary since 1993/1994, including those that have added services offered to beneficiaries and those that now have a greater volume of high-cost home health users, will likely experience the greatest impact under the new system.

The IPS reduces per visit cost limits 21 percent on average, and the HCFA projects that two-thirds of agencies will have costs in excess of those limits. The per beneficiary limit based on cost per patient in federal fiscal year 1994 requires home health agencies to focus on reducing costs per patient, through one or a combination of the following: reducing the number of visits provided, increasing the number of low-cost users, avoiding the admission of high-cost patients, or reducing costs per visit.

These changes could have a significant impact on agencies and the beneficiaries they serve. Some agencies could experience reductions in revenue and potential losses. Those agencies that cannot manage to make reductions may close. As a result of the per beneficiary limits, high-need/high-cost patients may have difficulty accessing services or experience reductions in service. Despite the need to reduce costs, agencies must also maintain quality. This will likely require the adoption of new utilization and care management protocols, as well as enhanced data capabilities, which carry increased costs that may not be reimbursable under the new limits.

REFERENCES

Bishop, C., & Skwara, K.C. (1993). Recent growth of Medicare home health. *Health Affairs, 12*(3), 95–110.

Cretin, S., & Worthman, L.G. (1986). *Alternative systems for case mix classification in health care financing.* Cooperative Agreement No. 99-C-98489/9-03. Prepared for the Health Care Financing Administration. Santa Monica, CA: Rand Corporation.

Fries, B.E., & Cooney, L.M. (1985). Resource utilization groups: A patient classification system for long term care. *Medical Care, 23*(2), 110–122.

Goldberg, H.B., & Schmitz, R.J. (1994). Contemplating home health PPS: Current patterns of Medicare service use. *Health Care Financing Review, 16*(1), 109–130.

Kenney, G.M. (1991). Understanding the effects of PPS on Medicare home health use. *Inquiry, 18,* 129–139.

Kenney, G.M., & Moon, M. (1997). *Reining in the growth in Medicare home health care.* New York: The Commonwealth Fund.

Leon, J., Neuman, P., & Paranet, S. (1997). *Understanding the growth in Medicare's home health expenditures.* Washington, DC: The Kaiser Family Foundation.

Proctor, E.K., Morrow-Howell, N., & Kaplan, S.J. (in press). The implementation of discharge plans for chronically ill elders discharged home. *Health & Social Work.*

Prospective Payment Assessment Commission. (1996). *Medicare and the American health care system: Report to Congress.* Washington, DC: Author.

Schneider, D.P., Fries, B.E., Foley, W.J., Desmond, M., & Gormley, W.J. (1988). Case mix for nursing home payment: Resource utilization groups, version II. *Health Care Financing Review,* (1988 Suppl.), 39–52.

Schore, J. (1994). *Patient, agency, and area characteristics associated with regional variation in the use of Medicare home health services.* Report prepared for the Health Care Financing Administration. Princeton, NJ: Mathematical Policy Research, Inc.

Shaughnessy, P.W., Schlenker, R.E., & Hittle, D.F. (1994). Home health care outcomes under capitated and fee-for-service payment. *Health Care Financing Review, 16*(1), 187–222.

Williams, B. (1994). Comparison of services among different types of home health agencies. *Medical Care, 32,* 1134–1152.

SUGGESTED READING

Brown, R., Bergeron, J., Clement, D., Hill, J., & Retchin, S. (1993). *The Medicare risk program for HMOs—The final summary report on findings from the evaluation.* Princeton, NJ: Mathematical Policy Research, Inc.

Kenney, G.M. (1993). Is access to home health care a problem in rural areas? *American Journal of Public Health, 83,* 412–414.

Kenney, G.M., & Dubay, L.C. (1992). Explaining area variation in the use of Medicare home health services. *Medical Care, 30,* 43–57.

Kenney, G.M., Rajan, S., & Socia, S. (1997). *Interactions between the Medicare and Medicaid home care programs: Insights from the states.* Urban Institute Working Paper.

Nyman, J.A., Sen, A., Chan, B.Y., & Commins, P.P. (1991). Urban/rural differences in home health patients and services. *The Gerontologist, 31,* 457–466.

Office of the Inspector General. (1995). *Variation among home health agencies in Medicare payments for home health services* (OEI-04-93-00260). Washington, DC: Author.

Scalzi, C.C., Zinn, J.S., Guifoyle, M.J., & Perdue, S.T. (1994). Medicare-certified home health services: National and regional supply in the 1980s. *American Journal of Public Health, 84*(10), 1646–1648.

Shaughnessy, P.W., et al. (1994). *A study to develop outcome-based quality measures for home health services:* Volume I: *Final report measuring outcomes of home health care.* Denver, CO: Center for Health Policy Research.

Swan, J.H., & Benjamin, A.E. (1990). Medicare home health utilization as a function of nursing home market factors. *Health Services Research, 25,* 479–500.

CHAPTER 10

Future Trends in Home Health Care

This chapter discusses some of the proposed future changes in home health care that may affect the practice of home health speech-language pathology. It is not intended to be all-inclusive, and, as with any predictions of the future, it is subject to change. However, the topics presented are areas that speech-language pathologists in home care should address.

INTRODUCTION

Over the past decade, those working in home health care have seen an increase in the acuity level of their patients. The length of stay in hospitals has become shorter and shorter, and home care providers deal with patients in the more acute stages of illness. In other words, home care providers are being asked to get patients better in a shorter period of time. This is quite a challenge to those individuals who work in home health care. Ultimately, the professionals working in home health care need to work together in a cohesive team to identify patients' needs more quickly and get the appropriate services to patients at the best time in recovery. If home health care professionals are able to accomplish this, they will maximize patient outcomes and minimize patients' need for hospitalization. This concept does not emphasize underutilization or overutilization but focuses on smart utilization. It is most important that speech-language pathologists point out to other team members the role that speech-language pathology plays in this concept of smart utilization. One of the greatest challenges facing speech-language pathologists in home health care is defining their role in the continuum of care. The clinician must be able to prove the impact of treatment on the patient's health.

CHANGING GOALS

One of the major goals that the speech-language pathologist wants to achieve in home health care is moving a patient from a state of dependence to some form of functional independence. To take this a step further, the continuum of care is not only for speech-language pathologists and their rehabilitative partners but for any discipline working with patients in the home care environment. The difficult task is being able to predict outcomes in a diverse patient population with very specific needs. The new changes in home health care from the federal and managed care perspective put pressure on clinicians to move away from any form of maintenance treatment or keeping people "on caseload" for any prolonged period of time. The goal now is to move patients out of the home care system, which ultimately will reduce the cost. Home health care patients now will not be seen for long periods of time. In the past, it was not uncommon for a speech-language pathologist to see a stroke patient for six to eight months. In today's marketplace, however, these treatment strategies are being looked at closely and more than likely will be markedly reduced. Clinicians who practice old methods of treating communication disorders, such as doing repetitive exercises, will not be able to sustain themselves in the upcoming home health care marketplace. The goals of the speech-language pathologist must be to educate the interdisciplinary care team in the role that communication plays in improving patients' health.

Chapter 2 addressed the current practice of medical services in home health care. At one time, practitioners from each discipline treated the patient, with little coordination of care. The pendulum is swinging toward establishing a more traditional care model, as was practiced in the early years of home health care. In the past 10 to 15 years, health care delivery in the home has become fragmented. One of the many reasons for this fragmentation is the visit-driven system that has characterized home health care since the early 1980s. When the quantity of visits is emphasized, there is little time for the individual disciplines to communicate with one another except through paper. One discipline did not know what the other was doing, and somewhere the patient was trapped in the middle. This type of care provision was confusing not only to the disciplines but also to patients and their families. So, the old way of providing home health care is not going to be good enough anymore. The federal mandates are now requiring home health professionals to increase their coordination by using other disciplines to the maximum and communicating effectively. So now home health care will be more of an interdisciplinary form of care with the nurse functioning as a case manager.

Interdisciplinary care means communication among and between the disciplines. Disciplines should be complementary to one another, and areas in which each discipline can assist in progressing other disciplines' goals should be defined. Most professional ideas of interdisciplinary care are really forms of transdisciplinary care. In transdisciplinary care, each individual discipline treats the patient, and someone, usually nursing services, coordinates the care in some fashion. In actuality, speech-language pathologists must ask themselves what they can do to help nursing to improve patients' health outcomes. This concept is more truly interdisciplinary care. The idea of interdisciplinary care is not that the speech-language pathologist would actually do nursing care or physical therapy but that the speech-language pathologist would provide modalities such as appropriate teaching methodologies, testing of cognition, and establishing modalities of learning that would assist the other disciplines to improve their patient outcomes.

PREPARING FOR CHANGES UNDER MANAGED CARE

Managed care is changing the way speech-language pathologists treat patients in home health care. To succeed in this new environment, clinicians can no longer rely solely on the skills and knowledge that helped them in the past. Professionals and patients need to understand the forces propelling managed care toward its final destination. These forces include economics, consumerism, science, and health care regulation.

Economic and consumer pressures combine to effect managed care. Consumers will no longer stand for exorbitant medical bills. Inexpensive, quality health care has attracted many older persons to relinquish their Medicare payment and benefits and align with managed care plans. Many managed care plans claim to be able to service these patients more cheaply and effectively.

This is where economic pressure comes into play. Competition among managed care organizations forces third-party payers to live up to their end of the deal at the risk of losing covered members to another managed care organization or to Medicare. The trend toward managed care forces speech-language pathologists to deliver an outcome for which the managed care organizations will pay and with which the patient can live. Speech-language pathologists have to change their treatment methodology because they will see patients for less time but still must maximize patient capabilities. Delivering all treatment modalities in a limited period of time is impossible; therefore, prioritizing goals has become a critical step in the overall treatment paradigm. To prioritize, the clinician needs to know outcome data related to the treatment.

The loss of treatment time causes clinicians to train family members earlier than before, depending on the cognitive skills of the patient. In addition, the family or patient caregiver will more than likely play a significant role in the provision of treatment. Clinicians will see that training families and caregivers, rather than using assistants, might be the most cost-effective measure. Certain goals may be pursued in the home by the same or other disciplines.

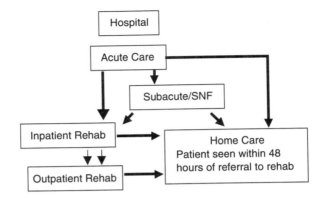

**CRITICAL TO GOOD CONTINUUM OF PATIENT CARE
FROM HOSPITAL TO HOME CARE**

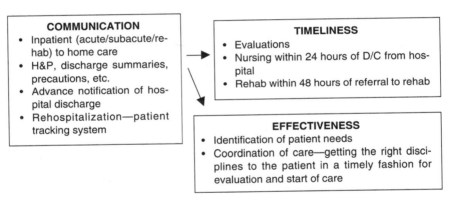

Figure 10–1 Continuum of Patient Care. Courtesy of Communication Concepts and Consulting, Inc., Birmingham, Alabama.

Another change fueling managed care comes from science. There is a lot of research about rehabilitation outcomes, and the results say more therapy is not necessarily better for patients. Many variables affect outcomes, however, and the results may not hold true in all cases. Treating a patient under Medicare for six weeks may not result in a better outcome than seeing a managed care beneficiary for two weeks. These findings are expediting the paradigm shift prompted by economic forces: Clinicians have to work smarter with less time and still achieve positive outcomes. The focus during therapy is on those items that will make a functional difference for the patient.

Home health care was never intended to be a long-term care program. The Conditions of Participation defined home health care as "intermittent skilled services," which shows that the emphasis in home health care from the beginning was short-term care. The major goal of home health care is to get the patient independent as quickly as possible. In this context, then, the federal government is only asking health care providers to administer the program as it was originally intended. So rehabilitation specialists must help improve patient health in a shorter period of time. The goal is to improve patient outcomes.

Another aspect of change is the patient's progress through the continuum of care. Figure 10–1 shows a schematic of the several ways patients go through the continuum, for example, from acute care inpatient to outpatient care or from acute care inpatient to home care. Some of these patients will go from acute care to subacute units at the hospital or at a skilled nursing facility and then on to inpatient or outpatient care, or from subacute to home care. And increasingly, patients are going from acute care hospitals directly home, a situation that may be due more to managed money rather than to managed care. It is going to be very important for all health professionals to look at the criteria so that a patient can be properly placed and obtain the best care available.

THE CHANGING ROLE OF THE SPEECH-LANGUAGE PATHOLOGIST

Recent changes in the home care environment have led speech-language pathologists to worry about their own well-being as well as the well-being of their patients. There is a lot of uncertainty in the air. Clinicians must become accustomed to change and be willing to act quickly and in an innovative manner to survive this changing environment. The interim payment system (IPS) is the reimbursement system of today, but this will change October 1, 1999, when home health agencies will be reimbursed under a prospective payment system. There will also be a 100-visit limit under Medicare Part A (after a three-day hospitalization or skilled nursing facility stay, a condition that will be phased in between 1999 and 2000). For the next several years, the focus will not be on technology and research but on budgets and costs.

Therapists need to explain the preventive nature and the cost-saving benefits of rehabilitative services, for example, why four more visits at this time could reduce the risk of falls, injury, or illness in the future. Speech-language pathologists may need to educate the nurse on the high risk of aspiration and the subsequent risk of pneumonia and possible hospitalization, which could be minimized by five treatment sessions to determine the appropriate texture of food and to train the caregivers in the appropriate care. Physical therapy can reduce the risk of falls and injury by training patients in basic safety techniques, determining appropriate assistive devices, and providing a home exercise program in just a couple of visits. Occupational therapy can train a patient or caregiver in activities of daily living and reduce the need for home health aide visits. And speech-language pathologists can provide cognitive training and reduce the need for continued nursing visits to educate the patient or caregiver in new medication regimens. These are but a few ways clinicians can begin to integrate their services in this changing environment. One of the most significant changes clinicians will see in the future will be the therapist in the role of educator. The therapist's role as educator will be to facilitate participation and compliance, educate nonlicensed staff, and educate families and patients.

Speech-language pathologists may also need to educate physicians and others who are not fully aware of the spectrum of services that speech-language pathologists provide. The following are some examples of the speech-language pathologist's role as an important part of the team:

- determining what factors are causing a functional deficit
- determining what the current functional deficits are and which impairments contributed to the patient's overall functional limitations
- determining which impairments can be remedied by treatment and which require compensatory training
- monitoring and adjusting treatments
- preventing problems or minimizing effects of degenerative diseases to promote quality of life
- ensuring safety in activities of daily living, mobility, dining, and eating

COMPUTERIZED OR AUTOMATED CLINICAL DOCUMENTATION

It is forecasted that the home care industry will invest more than $1.2 billion in information management technology by the year 2000 (Stern, 1996). A significant portion of these expenditures will involve computerized technical documentation systems, which offer the potential to reduce costs, streamline paperwork, and improve organizational performance.

The Documentation Process

Documentation has been cited as one of the most frustrating aspects of home health care (Lynch, 1994). Home care nurses are generally more satisfied than nurses in other practice settings, but they are almost unanimous in identifying documentation as the major source of dissatisfaction (Baldwin & Price, 1994). Federal regulations, accreditation standards, and reimbursement procedures dictate the critical data that must be recorded, and as a result documentation may account for up to 50 percent of the home care professional's time (Westra & Raup, 1995).

Home care documentation is essentially a paper-driven system, which contributes to the overall frustration of professionals working in the industry. Manual documentation is the established norm in health care and may be acceptable in institutional settings where the patient and clinical record are available at the same location. Home care, in contrast, is a movable industry, with care being provided at multiple locations. Clinical data, recorded at the site of care delivery, must be transported to the office for filing, and the staff must return to the office to access the clinical record. As a result, the paper-driven system can be cumbersome and time-consuming.

Manual documentation, although accepted, is not always effective in home care. The staff may provide high-quality care, but this is not necessarily reflected in the manual charting, which is often done after the fact. Clinicians have generally postponed charting to the end of the day, resulting in the loss of valuable information due to incomplete recall. In addition, the multitude of forms required to meet specific data collection requirements contributes to the duplication of entries and results in a lack of consistency. Each form stands independent of the others, making it difficult to monitor the patient's progress and promote coordination of care.

Computerization has been proposed as the solution to frustration with documentation. Initial attempts were limited to billing software, along with automated data entry to produce the plan of treatment. The growth and sophistication of claims submission packages simplified the billing process but did little to address the inadequacies associated with manual documentation. The industry as a whole is now moving toward computerized or automated documentation.

Documenting Functional Outcomes

Documented outcomes are essential in the managed care prospective payment environment. Clinicians must prove that what the patient is receiving (and what the insurance company is paying for) is actually making a difference. The need for such proof led to the development of the Outcome and Assessment Information Set (OASIS) and other functional outcome measures.

To achieve outcomes, clinicians must have a standardized way of delivering the skills needed by the patient to be functionally independent. Therefore, clinicians must develop critical pathways or care maps. Critical pathways ensure that what Therapist A does will have the same impact as what Therapist B would do in the same circumstance. By using the critical pathway and then measuring the outcome achieved, the case manager can ensure that the therapy is both effective and cost efficient.

In a capitated system (per patient limit per year), the emphasis will be on short lengths of stays and few visits. There will also be an emphasis on preventing future admissions to the agency, as there will be no additional money for second or third admissions for the same diagnosis. Home health agencies should realize that rehabilitative services will enable them to reach this goal.

Interdisciplinary care is and will be an important aspect of patient care. All disciplines will have to be cross-trained (multiskilled) to a certain extent. To reduce the total number of visits, therapists may need to document vital signs in the chart, or the aide may have to help with exercises for activities of daily living. Communication among disciplines is of utmost importance.

PROPOSED CHANGES IN THE CONDITIONS OF PARTICIPATION

In addition to the changes discussed previously, the Health Care Financing Administration (HCFA) is proposing changes in the Conditions of Participation for home care agencies. These proposed changes were published in the *Federal Register* in August 1998. Every clinician should become familiar with the Conditions of Participation. This section briefly reviews the proposed changes to the Conditions of Participation and their possible effects on the practice of speech-language pathology. All the proposed changes in the Conditions of Participation for home health agencies are not presented, but the information most critical to speech-language pathologists is included. All clinical personnel are encouraged to monitor these new conditions and anticipated publication in the *Federal Register*.

On March 10, 1997, the HCFA released the proposed revision of the Conditions of Participation for home health agencies. These revisions reflect a new focus on improving the home health agency's performance. The HCFA has proposed a restructuring of the Conditions of Participation, revising the current regulations, incorporating new concepts, and deleting some information that is no longer relevant. There are currently 12 conditions and 32 standards. The proposed regulations include 9 conditions and 42 standards. The revised regulations include 4 core conditions:

1. patient rights
2. comprehensive assessment of patients
3. care planning and coordination of services
4. quality assessment and performance improvement

The conditions on comprehensive assessment include mandatory use of the OASIS instrument.

Patient Rights

In addition to the already established guidelines for home patient rights, the patient now must also be informed about expected outcomes of treatment and barriers to treatment. Expected outcomes are patient goals and objectives. Barriers to treatment may include lack of family and emotional support, communication education deficits, lack of financial resources, or lack of nutrition. The HCFA's emphasis is on interdisciplinary care. Clinicians will have to identify their goals and objectives up front. Clinicians will have to become more efficient at differential diagnosis on the initial visit. In addition, the clinician will have to obtain a lot of information in a short period of time. Identifying patient goals and objectives and any barriers to treatment will be done on the initial assessment. Making referrals to the appropriate disciplines will need to be not only accurate but timely.

Care Planning and Coordination

There are proposed new changes to the review and revision of the plan of care. A plan of care must be reviewed and updated at least every 62 days.

Staff must promptly alert the physician if measurable outcomes are not being achieved. The home health agency must reassess and document the patient's response to current medical and environmental situations (including barriers to care), and implement a physician's revised plan of care as needed. The revised plan of care must relate to the updated comprehensive assessment (OASIS). Coordination of care must be interdisciplinary, based on patient needs and barriers to care, and include the patient and family and the physician (for relevant medical issues).

FRAUD AND ABUSE INITIATIVES

Operation Restore Trust

Operation Restore Trust is an effort by the Department of Health and Human Services to combat health care fraud, waste, and abuse. The project started in the five states (California, Florida, Illinois, New York, and Texas) that have nearly 40 percent of all Medicare and Medicaid beneficiaries and the highest Medicare expenditures. The initial two-year Operation Restore Trust demonstration project, which focused on home health agencies, nursing homes, durable medical equipment suppliers, and hospices, ended in March 1997. Operation Restore Trust has since been expanded to include 12 new targeted states—Arizona, Colorado, Georgia, Louisiana, Massachusetts, Missouri, New Jersey, Ohio, Pennsylvania, Tennessee, Virginia, and Washington—in addition to the original five and to target additional providers, including psychiatric hospitals and other mental health providers, laboratories, and ancillary nursing home services such as physical therapy.

The Operation Restore Trust project is an interdisciplinary partnership composed of the Department of Health and Human Services Office of the Inspector General, HCFA, and Administration on Aging; the Department of Justice; U.S. Attorneys Offices, HCFA contractors (carriers and intermediaries) and contractor fraud unit; Medicaid fraud control units; state surveyors; state long-term care ombudsmen; and state attorneys general. Working together, these agencies educated the health care industry and the public, including Medicare beneficiaries and Medicaid recipients, on types of activities and behaviors that indicate fraudulent or abusive activity. An individual suspicious of provider activities can write the Office of the Inspector General or call a hotline number set up specifically for this purpose, or the individual can report the suspicious conduct directly to the Department of Justice, the local U.S. Attorneys Office, the state attorney general, the intermediary or carrier, or the state Medicaid fraud control units. When warranted, an investigation of the provider would ensue, which may be performed by the intermediary or carrier's fraud unit, the Office of the Inspector General's investigators and/or auditors, the Department of Justice and its investigators (including agents with the Federal Bureau of Investigation), and the state. Investigations could lead to civil lawsuits against the provider, a criminal indictment, civil and/or criminal settlement, or the closing of the case.

The Wedge Project

The Wedge Project is an Operation Restore Trust–type project started by the HCFA, which decided to directly pursue all waste and abuse in high-utilization home health agencies. The HCFA started Wedge with $3.5 million allocated to the agency by the Health Insurance Portability and Accountability Act of 1996, and the project's name is a reference to the fact that the money came from a slice of the bill that was not specifically allocated for any purpose. States involved in the Wedge Project were chosen on the basis of proposals submitted by the states to the HCFA. While Operation Restore Trust focused on high-volume states, the Wedge Project focuses on states with high rates of utilization for individual providers.

The Wedge Project is also multidisciplinary, but with a smaller team than that of Operation Restore Trust. The Wedge Project, a joint effort by the HCFA, state surveyors, and fiscal intermediaries, is essentially the merging of fraud investigations with routine state surveys of compliance with the Medicare Conditions of Participation. The states engaged in Wedge are looking at different providers and conducting their audits differently, although a common theme is that audits typically involve 15 claims per provider for a two-month period.

OTHER FEDERAL REIMBURSEMENT CHANGES

Prospective Payment Provision

The prospective payment provision requires the Secretary of the Department of Health and Human Services to establish a prospective payment system for home health and to implement the system beginning October 1, 1999. All services covered and paid on a reasonable cost basis at the time of enactment of this section, including medical supplies, are required to be paid on a prospective basis. The provision allows the Secretary a transition of up to four years to implement the prospective payment system. During this time, a portion of the payment would be based on agency-specific cost, but the aggregate payments cannot be more than they would have been if there was no transition.

The Secretary is authorized to consider the following elements in the prospective payment system: (1) an appropriate unit of service and the number of visits provided within that unit, (2) potential changes in the mix of services provided within that unit and their costs, and (3) a general system design that provides for continued access to quality services.

The Secretary would compute a standard prospective payment amount that would initially be based on the most current audited cost report data available. For fiscal year 2000, payment amounts under the prospective payment system are to be computed so that the total payments would equal amounts that would have been paid had no prospective payment system been in effect. If the Secretary is unable to implement a prospective payment system by October 1, 1999, the legislation requires that the cost limits and per beneficiary limits in effect September 30, 1999, be reduced by 15 percent.

Reduction in Cost Limits

Under the law, limits for individual home care services are set at 112 percent of the mean labor-related and nonlabor per visit costs for free-standing agencies. The limits are effective for cost reporting periods beginning on or after July 1 of a given year and ending June 30 of the following year.

Under the recent legislative change, before the prospective payment system is implemented, the cost limits are reduced to 105 percent of the national median of labor-related and nonlabor costs for free-standing home care agencies, effective for cost reporting periods beginning October 1, 1997.

Medicare Salary Equivalency

Steady and steep increases in speech-language pathology and occupational therapy cost-based charges by some rehabilitation service contractors was the main purpose for the HCFA's decision to implement salary equivalency per hour limits.

The HCFA acknowledged in a March 1997 *Federal Register* proposal that one reason contractors have boosted charges for speech-language pathology and occupational therapy service is to compensate for low physical therapy salary equivalency reimbursement limits.

Medicare law permits salary equivalency limits to apply when any health care facility, agency, or clinic (not a medical group) furnishes "under arrangements" speech-language pathology, occupational therapy, physical therapy, or other therapy services. On January 30, 1998, the much-anticipated rule for Medicare salary equivalency rates for rehabilitation professions was released. The final speech-language pathology national hourly salary equivalency guideline is $46.23. The final national rates for occupational therapy and physical therapy are $48.06 and $50.65, respectively. The salary equivalency guidelines are based on equivalency to actual salaries in hospitals, nursing homes, and other settings. Levels of professional education and other qualifications were not considered in the analysis.

ANTICIPATED EFFECTS

The HCFA states that the following expected effects will result in a better functioning, more efficient health care system:

- Efficiently run rehabilitation companies may cut expenses and become more efficient, as is happening in much of the rest of the economy.
- More efficient companies may expand or enter the market, picking up the therapy services volume that less efficient suppliers may leave unserved.
- Overhead is a likely candidate for expense reduction.
- A deceleration in wage increases for workers with exceedingly high compensation levels will continue until wages are roughly comparable for each therapy type.
- Therapists who lose their jobs because of curtailed contractual services by rehabilitation companies may
  - work for rehabilitation agencies that bill Medicare directly
  - change employers to those efficiently run companies that expand their contracted services
  - become self-employed and contract directly with facilities

CONCLUSION

There are many changes and challenges facing the home care speech-language pathologist. Changes in practice patterns, reimbursement, and accountability are expected in the future. The information provided in this chapter was current at the time the text was printed, but clinicians should keep abreast of upcoming changes.

REFERENCES

Baldwin, D., & Price, S. (1994). Work excitement: The energizer of home healthcare nursing. *Journal of Nursing Administration, 24*, 37–42.

Lynch, S. (1994). Job satisfaction of home health nurses. *Home Healthcare Nurse, 12*, 21–28

Stern, E. (1996). Key management information strategies. *Remington Report, 4*, 10–13.

Westra, B., & Raup, G. (1995). Computerized charting: An essential tool for survival. *Caring, 15*, 52–57.

SUGGESTED READING

American Speech-Language-Hearing Association. (1998). Medicare salary equivalency. *ASHA Bulletin,* February 2.

Antone, T.V., & Sylvia, L.M. (1997, October). *How your agency can survive an ORT or Wedge investigation.* Paper presented at the American Federation of Home Health Agencies Convention, Las Vegas, NV.

Levy, S. (1997, October). *Get ready for the reimbursement revolution: Many ways to cut your costs.* Paper presented at the American Federation of Home Health Agencies Convention, Las Vegas, NV.

Physician Certification and Plan of Treatment Requirements

(Medicare—Code of Federal Regulations, Title 42)

PLAN OF TREATMENT REQUIREMENTS

§410.61 Plan of Treatment Requirements for Outpatient Physical Therapy and Speech Pathology Services

(a) *Basic requirement.* Outpatient physical therapy services (including services furnished by a qualified physical therapist in independent practice), and outpatient speech pathology services must be furnished under a written plan of treatment that meets the requirements of paragraphs (b) through (e) of this section.

(b) *Establishment of the plan.* The plan is established before treatment is begun by one of the following:*

(1) A physician.

(2) A physical therapist who will furnish the physical therapy services.

(3) A speech pathologist who will furnish the speech pathology services.

(c) *Content of the plan.* The plan prescribes the type, amount, frequency, and duration of the physical therapy or speech pathology services to be furnished to the individual, and indicates the diagnosis and anticipated goals.

(d) *Changes in the plan.* Any changes in the plan—

(1) Are made in writing and signed by one of the following:

(i) The physician or the physical therapist or speech pathologist who furnishes the services.

---

*Before January 1981, only a physician could establish a plan of treatment for physical therapy or speech pathology services. Speech pathologists were authorized to establish a plan effective January 1, 1981; physical therapists, effective July 18, 1984.

Source: Reprinted from *Code of Federal Regulations, Title 42,* Medicare.

(ii) A registered professional nurse or a staff physician, in accordance with oral orders from the physician, physical therapist, or speech pathologist who furnishes the services.

(2) The changes are incorporated in the plan immediately.

(e) *Review of the plan.* (1) The physician reviews the plan as often as the individual's condition requires, but at least every 30 days.

(2) Each review is dated and signed by the physician who performs it.

[53 FR 6638, Mar. 2, 1988; 53 FR 12945, Apr. 20, 1988, as amended at 54 FR 38680, Sept. 20, 1989; 54 FR 46614, Nov. 6, 1989; Redesignated at 56 FR 8854, Mar. 1, 1991; 56 FR 23022, May 20, 1991]

§410.62 Outpatient Speech Pathology Services: Conditions and Exclusions

(a) *Basic rule.* Medicare Part B pays for outpatient speech pathology services if they meet the following conditions:

(1) They are furnished to a beneficiary while he or she is under the care of a physician who is a doctor of medicine or osteopathy.

(2) They are furnished under a written plan of treatment that—

(i) Is established by a physician or, effective January 1, 1982, by either a physician or the speech pathologist who will provide the services to the particular individual;

(ii) Is periodically reviewed by a physician; and

(iii) Meets the requirements of §410.63.

(3) They are furnished by a provider or by others under arrangements with, and under the supervision of, a provider.

(b) *Outpatient speech pathology services to certain inpatients of a hospital, RPCH, or SNF.* Medicare Part B pays for outpatient speech pathology services furnished to an inpatient of a hospital, RPCH, or SNF who requires them but has exhausted or is otherwise ineligible for benefit days under Medicare Part A.

(c) *Excluded services.* No service is included as an outpatient speech pathology service if it would not be included as an inpatient hospital service if furnished to a hospital or RPCH inpatient.

[(b) and (c) were revised May 26, 1993 to include rural primary care hospitals (RPCHs).]

[51 FR 41339, Nov. 14, 1986, as amended at 53 FR 6648, Mar. 2, 1988; 56 FR 8852, Mar. 1, 1991; 56 FR 23022, May 20, 1991]

PHYSICIAN CERTIFICATION REQUIREMENTS

§424.10 Purpose and Scope

(a) *Purpose.* The physician is the key figure in determining utilization of health services furnished by providers. The physician decides upon admissions, orders tests, drugs, and treatments, and determines the length of stay. Accordingly, sections 1814(a)(2) and (3) and 1835(a)(2) of the Act establish as a condition for Medicare payment that a physician certify the necessity of the services and, in some instances, recertify the continued need for those services.

(b) *Scope.* This subpart sets forth the timing, content, and signature requirements for physician certification and recertification with respect to certain Medicare services furnished by providers.

[53 FR 6635, Mar. 2, 1988; 53 FR 12945, Apr. 20, 1988; 56 FR 8853, Mar. 1, 1991]

§424.11 General Procedures

(a) *Responsibility of the provider.* The provider must—

(1) Obtain the required certification and recertification statements;

(2) Keep them on file for verification by the intermediary, if necessary; and

(3) Certify, on the appropriate billing form, that the statements have been obtained and are on file.

(b) *Obtaining the certification and recertification statements.* No specific procedures or forms are required for certification and recertification statements. The provider may adopt any method that permits verification. The certification and recertification statements may be entered on forms, notes, or records that a physician signs, or on a special separate form. Except as provided in paragraph (d) of this section for delayed certifications, there must be a separate signed statement for each certification or recertification.

(c) *Required information.* The succeeding sections of this subpart set forth specific information required for different types of services. If that information is contained in other provider records, such as physicians' progress notes, it need not be repeated. It will suffice for the statement to indicate where the information is to be found.

(d) *Timeliness.* (1) The succeeding sections of this subpart also specify the time frames for certifications and for initial and subsequent recertifications.

(2) A hospital or SNF may provide for obtaining a certification or recertification earlier than required by these regulations, or vary the time frame (within the prescribed outer limits) for different diagnostic or clinical categories.

(3) Delayed certification and recertification statements are acceptable when there is a legitimate reason for delay. (For instance, the patient was unaware of his or her entitlement when he or she was treated.) Delayed certification and recertification statements must include an explanation of the reason for the delay.

(4) A delayed certification may be included with one or more recertifications on a single signed statement.

(e) *Limitation on authorization to sign statements.* A physician certification or recertification statement may be signed only by one of the following:

(1) A physician who is a doctor of medicine or osteopathy.

(2) A dentist in the circumstances specified in §424.13(c).

(3) A doctor of podiatric medicine if his or her certification is consistent with the functions he or she is authorized to perform under State law.

[53 FR 6634, Mar. 2, 1968, as amended at 56 FR 8845, Mar. 1, 1991]

§424.13 Requirements for Inpatient Services of Hospitals Other Than Psychiatric Hospitals

(a) *Content of certification and recertification.* Medicare Part A pays for inpatient hospital services of hospitals other than psychiatric hospitals only if a physician certifies and recertifies the following:

(1) The reasons for either—

(i) Continued hospitalization of the patient for medical treatment or medically required inpatient diagnostic study; or

(ii) Special or unusual services for cost outlier cases (under the prospective payment system set forth in subpart F of part 412 of this chapter).

(2) The estimated time the patient will need to remain in the hospital.

(3) The plans for posthospital care, if appropriate.

(b) *Certification of need for hospitalization when a SNF bed is not available.* (1) A physician may certify or recertify need for continued hospitalization if the physician finds that the patient could receive proper treatment in a SNF but no bed is available in a participating SNF.

(2) If this is the basis for the physician's certification or recertification, the required statement must so indicate; and the physician is expected to continue efforts to place the patient in a participating SNF as soon as a bed becomes available.

(c) *Signatures.* (1) *Basic rule.* Except as specified in paragraph (c)(2) of this section, certifications and recertifications must be signed by the physician responsible for the case, or by another physician who has knowledge of the case and who is authorized to do so by the responsible physician or by the hospital's medical staff.

(2) *Exception.* If the intermediary requests certification of the need to admit a patient in connection with dental procedures, because his or her underlying medi-

cal condition and clinical status or the severity of the dental procedures require[s] hospitalization, that certification may be signed by the dentist caring for the patient.

(d) *Timing of certifications and recertifications: Cases not subject to the prospective payment system* (PPS). (1) For cases that are not subject to PPS, certification is required no later than as of the 12th day of hospitalization. A hospital may, at its option, provide for the certification to be made earlier, or it may vary the timing of the certification within the 12-day period by diagnostic or clinical categories.

(2) The first recertification is required no later than as of the 18th day of hospitalization.

(3) Subsequent recertifications are required at intervals established by the UR committee (on a case-by-case basis if it so chooses), but no less frequently than every 30 days.

(e) *Timing of certification and recertification: Cases subject to PPS.* For cases subject to PPS, certification is required as follows:

(1) For day-outlier cases, certification is required no later than one day after the hospital reasonably assumes that the case meets the outlier criteria, established in accordance with §412.80(a)(1)(i) of this chapter, or no later than 20 days into the hospital stay, whichever is earlier. The first and subsequent recertifications are required at intervals established by the UR committee (on a case-by-case basis if it so chooses) but not less frequently than every 30 days.

(2) For cost-outlier cases, certification is required no later than the date on which the hospital requests cost outlier payment or 20 days into the hospital stay, whichever is earlier. If possible, certification must be made before the hospital incurs costs for which it will seek cost outlier payment. In cost outlier cases, the first and subsequent recertifications are required at intervals established by the UR committee (on a case-by-case basis if it so chooses).

(f) *Recertification requirement fulfilled by utilization review.* (1) At the hospital's option, extended stay review by its UR committee may take the place of the second and subsequent physician recertifications required for cases not subject to PPS and for PPS day-outlier cases.

(2) A utilization review that is used to fulfill the recertification requirement is considered timely if performed no later than the seventh day after the day the physician recertification would have been required. The next physician recertification would need to be made no later than the 30th day following such review; if review by the UR committee took the place of this physician recertification, the review could be performed as late as the seventh day following the 30th day.

(g) *Description of procedures.* The hospital must have available on file a written description that specifies the time schedule for certifications and recertifications, and indicates whether utilization review of long-stay cases fulfills the requirement for second and subsequent recertifications of all cases not subject to PPS and of PPS day outlier cases.

§424.20 Requirements for Posthospital SNF Care

Medicare Part A pays for posthospital SNF care furnished by a SNF or a hospital with a swing-bed approval only if a physician certifies and recertifies the need for services consistent with the content of paragraph (a) or (c) of this section, as appropriate.

(a) *Content of certification*—(1) *General requirements.* (i) Posthospital SNF care is or was required because the individual needs or needed on a daily basis skilled nursing care (furnished directly by or requiring the supervision of skilled nursing personnel) or other skilled rehabilitation services that, as a practical matter, can only be provided in a SNF or a swing-bed hospital on an inpatient basis; and

(ii) The SNF care is or was needed for a condition for which the individual received inpatient care in a participating hospital or a qualified hospital, as defined in §409.3 of this chapter.

(2) *Special requirement: A swing-bed hospital with more than 49 beds (but fewer than 100) that does not transfer a swing-bed patient to a SNF within 5 days of the availability date.* Transfer of the extended care patient to the SNF is not medically appropriate.

(b) *Timing of certification*—(1) *General rule.* The certification must be obtained at the time of admission or as soon thereafter as is reasonable and practicable.

(2) *Special rules for certain swing-bed hospitals.* For swing-bed hospitals with more than 49 beds that are approved after March 31, 1988, the extended care patient's physician has 5 days (excluding weekends and holidays) beginning on the availability date as defined in §413.114(b), to certify that the transfer of the extended care patient is not medically appropriate.

(c) *Content of recertifications.* (1) The reasons for the continued need for posthospital SNF care;

(2) The estimated time the individual will need to remain in the SNF;

(3) Plans for home care, if any; and

(4) If appropriate, the fact that continued services are needed for a condition that arose after admission to the SNF and while the individual was still under treatment for the condition for which he or she had received inpatient hospital services.

(d) *Timing of recertifications.* (1) The first recertification is required no later than the 14th day of posthospital SNF care.

(2) Subsequent recertifications are required at least every 30 days after the first recertification.

(e) *Signature*. Certification and recertification statements may be signed by the physician responsible for the case or, with his or her authorization, by a physician on the SNF staff or a physician who is available in case of an emergency and has knowledge of the case.

(f) *Recertification requirement fulfilled by utilization review*. A SNF may substitute utilization review of extended stay cases for the second and subsequent recertifications, if it includes this procedure in its utilization review plan.

(g) *Description of procedures*. The SNF must have available on file a written description that specifies the certification and recertification time schedule and indicates whether utilization review is used as an alternative to the second and subsequent recertifications.

[53 FR 6634, Mar. 2, 1988, as amended at 54 FR 37275, Sept. 7, 1989]

§424.22 Requirements for Home Health Services

Medicare Part A or Part B pays for home health services only if a physician certifies and recertifies the content specified in paragraphs (a)(1) and (b)(2) of this section, as appropriate.

(a) *Certification*—(1) *Content of certification*. As a condition for payment of home health services under Medicare Part A or Medicare Part B, a physician must certify as follows:

(i) The individual needs or needed intermittent skilled nursing care, or physical or speech therapy, or (for the period from July through November 30, 1981) occupational therapy.

(ii) Home health services were required because the individual was confined to the home except when receiving outpatient services.

(iii) A plan for furnishing the services has been established and is periodically reviewed by a physician who is a doctor of medicine, osteopathy, or podiatric medicine, and who is not precluded from performing this function under paragraph (d) of this section. (A doctor of podiatric medicine may perform only plan of treatment functions that are consistent with the functions he or she is authorized to perform under State law.)

(iv) The services were furnished while the individual was under the care of a physician who is a doctor of medicine, osteopathy, or podiatric medicine.*

---

* As a condition of Medicare Part A payment for home health services furnished before July 1981, the physician was also required to certify that the services were needed for a condition for which the individual had received inpatient hospital or SNF services.

(2) *Timing and signature.* The certification of need for home health services must be obtained at the time the plan of treatment is established or as soon thereafter as possible and must be signed by the physician who establishes the plan.

(b) *Recertification*—(1) *Timing and signature of recertification.* Recertification is required at least every 2 months, preferably at the time the plan is reviewed, and must be signed by the physician who reviews the plan.

(2) *Content and basis of recertification.* The recertification statement must indicate the continuing need for services and estimate how much longer the services will be required. Need for occupational therapy may be the basis for continuing services that were initiated because the individual needed skilled nursing care or physical or speech therapy.

(c) [Reserved]

(d) *Limitations on the performance of certification and plan of treatment functions*—(1) *Basic rule.* Beginning November 26, 1982, and except as provided in paragraph (e) of this section, need for home health services to be provided by an HHA may not be certified or recertified, and a plan of treatment may not be established and reviewed, by any physician who has a significant ownership interest in, or a significant financial or contractual relationship with, that HHA.

(2) *Significant ownership interest.* A physician is considered to have a significant ownership interest in an HHA if he or she—

(i) Has a direct or indirect ownership interest of 5 percent or more in the capital, the stock, or the profits of the home health agency; or

(ii) Has an ownership interest of 5 percent or more in any mortgage, deed of trust, note, or other obligation that is secured by the agency, if that interest equals 5 percent or more of the agency's assets.

(3) *Significant financial or contractual relationship.* Beginning November 26, 1982, a physician is considered to have a significant financial or contractual relationship with an HHA if he or she—

(i) Receives any compensation as an officer or director of the HHA; or

(ii) Has direct or indirect business transactions with the HHA that, in any fiscal year, amount to more than $25,000 or 5 percent of the agency's total operating expenses, whichever is less. Business transactions means contracts, agreements, purchase orders, or leases to obtain services, supplies, equipment, and space and, after August 29, 1986, salaried employment.

(4) *Exemption of uncompensated officer or director.* A physician who serves as an uncompensated officer or director of an HHA is not precluded from performing physician certification and plan of treatment functions for that HHA.

(e) *Exceptions to limitations.*—(1) *Exceptions for governmental entities.* The limitations of paragraph (d) of this section do not apply to an HHA that is operated by a Federal, State, or local governmental authority.

(2) *Exception for sole community HHAs.* The limitations of paragraph (d) of this section do not apply on or after the date on which the HHA is classified as a sole

community HHA in accordance with paragraphs (f) and (g) of this section.

(f) *Procedures for classification as a sole community HHA.* (1) The HHA must submit to its intermediary a request for classification, showing that it meets the conditions of paragraph (g) of this section.

(2) The intermediary reviews the request and sends the request, with its recommendations, to HCFA.

(3) HCFA reviews the request and the intermediary's recommendation and forwards its approval or disapproval to the intermediary

(4) An approved classification as sole community HHA remains in effect without need for reapproval unless there is a change in the circumstances under which the classification was approved.

(g) *Basis for classification as a sole community HHA.* HCFA approves a classification as a sole community HHA only if the HHA designates a particular area and shows that no other HHA provides services within that area.

[53 FR 6638, Mar. 2, 1988; 53 FR 12945, Apr. 20, 1988; 56 FR 8845, Mar. 1, 1991]

§424.24 Requirements for Medical and Other Health Services Furnished by Providers under Medicare Part B.

(a) *Exempted services.* Certification is not required for the following: (1) Hospital services and supplies incident to physicians' services furnished to outpatients. The exemption applies to drugs and biologicals that cannot be self-administered, but not to partial hospitalization services, as set forth in paragraph (e) of this section.

(2) Outpatient hospital diagnostic services, including necessary drugs and biologicals, ordinarily furnished or arranged for by a hospital for the purpose of diagnostic study.

(b) *General rule.* Medicare Part B pays for medical and other health services furnished by providers (and not exempted under paragraph (a) of this section) only if a physician certifies the content specified in paragraph (c)(1), (c)(4) or (e)(1) of this section, as appropriate.

(c) *Outpatient physical therapy and speech pathology services*—(1) *Content of certification.* (i) The individual needs, or needed, physical therapy or speech pathology services.

(ii) The services were furnished while the individual was under the care of a physician. (For physical therapy services furnished after July 17, 1984, the physician may be a doctor of podiatric medicine, provided the services are consistent with the functions he or she is authorized to perform under State law.)

(iii) The services were furnished under a plan of treatment that meets the requirements of §424.25.

(2) *Timing.* The certification statement must be obtained at the time the plan of treatment is established, or as soon thereafter as possible.

(3) *Signature.* (i) If the plan of treatment is established by a physician, the certification must be signed by that physician.

(ii) If the plan of treatment is established by a physical therapist or speech pathologist, the certification must be signed by a physician who has knowledge of the case.

(4) *Recertification*—(i) *Timing.* Recertification statements are required at least every 30 days and must be signed by the physician who reviews the plan of treatment.

(ii) *Content.* The continuing need for physical therapy or speech pathology services and an estimate of how much longer the services will be needed.

(d) [Reserved]

(e) *Partial hospitalization services: Content of certification and plan of treatment requirements*—(1) *Content of certification.* (i) The individual would require inpatient psychiatric care if the partial hospitalization services were not provided.

(ii) The services are or were furnished while the individual was under the care of a physician.

(iii) The services were furnished under a written plan of treatment that meets the requirements of paragraph (e)(2) of this section.

(2) *Plan of treatment requirements.* (i) The plan is an individualized plan that is established and is periodically reviewed by a physician in consultation with appropriate staff participating in the program, and that sets forth—

(A) The physician's diagnosis;

(B) The type, amount, duration, and frequency of the services; and

(C) The treatment goals under the plan.

(ii) The physician determines the frequency and duration of the services taking into account accepted norms of medical practice and a reasonable expectation of improvement in the patient's condition.

(f) *All other covered medical and other health services furnished by providers.*—(1) *Content of certification.* The services were medically necessary.

(2) *Signature.* The certificate must be signed by a physician who has knowledge of the case.

(3) *Timing.* The physician may provide certification at the time the services are furnished or, if services are provided on a continuing basis, either at the beginning or at the end of a series of visits.

(4) *Recertification.* Recertification of continued need for services is not required.

[53 FR 6638, Mar. 2, 1988; 53 FR 12945, Apr. 20, 1988; 56 FR 8845, Mar. 1, 1991]

§424.25 "Plan of Treatment Requirements for Outpatient Physical Therapy and Speech Pathology Services"

[This section has been redesignated as §410.61.]

§424.27 Requirements for Comprehensive Outpatient Rehabilitation Facility (CORF) Services

Medicare Part B pays for CORF services only if a physician certifies, and the facility physician recertifies, the content specified in paragraphs (a) and (b)(2) of this section, as appropriate.

(a) *Certification: Content.* (1) The services were required because the individual needed skilled rehabilitation services;

(2) The services were furnished while the individual was under the care of a physician; and

(3) A written plan of treatment has been established and is reviewed periodically by a physician.

(b) *Recertification*—(1) *Timing.* Recertification is required at least every 60 days, based on review by a facility physician who, when appropriate, consults with the professional personnel who furnish the services.

(2) *Content.* (i) The plan is being followed;

(ii) The patient is making progress in attaining the rehabilitation goals; and

(iii) The treatment is not having any harmful effect on the patient.

[53 FR 6634, Mar. 2, 1988.]

APPENDIX B

Generic Referral Form

GENERIC HOME HEALTH AGENCY REFERRAL FORM

Patient Name _____

Address _____ Apt # _____

City/State/ZIP _____

Phone _____ DOB _____ Sex _____

Primary Diagnosis _____ Onset Date _____

Secondary Diagnosis/Onset _____

Surgical Procedures/Dates _____

Medications _____

Physician _____ Phone_____

Address _____

Primary Caregiver _____ Relationship _____

Home Phone _____ Work Phone _____

Contact Name _____ Relationship _____

Home Phone _____ Work Phone _____

Last Hospital Stay from Date _____ to Date _____

Hospital Name _____ Hospital # _____

Payer Source/# _____

Referral Source _____ Telephone # _____

305

SN: ❏ EVAL
   ❏ VITAL SIGNS, CV, CP, TEMP
   ❏ OBSV BOWEL/ BLADDER STATUS
   ❏ NUTR/FLUID BAL
   ❏ MEDICATION
   ❏ CHECK WEIGHT
   ❏ CHECK BLOOD SUGAR
   ❏ DRESSING CHANGE
   ❏ PREFILL SYRINGE
   ❏ PAIN CONTROL
   ❏ CHECK S/S INF/HEAL
   ❏ CHECK NEURO STATUS
   ❏ OSTOMY CARE
   ❏ LAB WORK

❏ CATH CARE
❏ ADM IV/IM MEDS
❏ _____
FREQ: _____

AIDE: _____

SW: _____

ST: ❏ EVAL/TX
   ❏ LANG DIS TX
   ❏ DYSPHAGIA TX
   ❏ DYSPHASIA TX
   ❏ COGN RETRAIN
   ❏ _____
FREQ: _____

OT: ❏ EVAL/TX
   ❏ ADL RETRAIN
   ❏ STRENGTHENING
   ❏ ROM _____
   ❏ FINE MOTOR
   ❏ PERCEPT MOTOR
   ❏ MUSCLE RE-EDUCATION

❏ ADAPT EQUIPMENT
❏ HOME ASSESS
❏ _____
FREQ:
_____

PT: ❏ EVAL/TX
   ❏ ROM
   ❏ STRENGTHENING
   ❏ TRANSFERS
   ❏ GAIT TRAINING
   ❏ HEP
   ❏ ULTRASOUND
   ❏ SAFETY CHECK
   ❏ HOME ASSESS
   ❏ _____
FREQ:
WBS   _____
      _____

Remarks/Instructions: _____
_____
_____
_____
_____

Signature _____ Date _____

Service Codes for HCFA Forms 485 and 486

TREATMENT CODES FOR PROFESSIONAL SERVICES REQUIRED

Skilled Nursing

A1* Skilled Observation and Assessment (Inc. V.S., response to med., etc.)
A2   Foley Insertion
A3   Bladder Instillation
A4* Open Wound Care/Dressing
A5* Decubitus Care (partial tissue loss with signs of infection or full thickness tissue loss, etc.)
A6* Venipuncture
A7* Restorative Nursing
A8   Post Cataract Care
A9   Bowel/Bladder Training
A10 Chest Physio (Inc. postural drainage)
A11 Adm. of Vitamin B_{12}
A12 Adm. Insulin
A13 Adm. Other Im/Subq.
A14 Adm. IV/s/Clysis
A15 Teach Ostomy or Ileo Conduit Care
A16 Teach Nasogastric Feeding
A17 Reinsertion Nasogastric Feeding Tube
A18 Teach Gastrostomy Feeding

*Code that requires a more extensive descriptive narrative for physician's orders.

Source: Adapted from HIM-11, Health Care Financing Administration.

A19   Teach Parenteral Nutrition
A20   Teach Care of Trach
A21   Adm. Care of Trach
A22* Teach Inhalation Rx
A23* Adm. Inhalation Rx
A24   Teach Adm. of Injection
A25   Teach Diabetic Care
A26   Disimpaction/F.U. Enema
A27* Other (Spec. under Orders)
A28* Wound Care/Dressing—Closed Incision/Suture Line
A29* Decubitus Care (Other than A5)
A30   Teaching Care of Any Indwelling Catheter
A31   Management and Evaluation of Patient Care Plan
A32* Teaching and Training (other) (spec. under order)

Physical Therapy

B1   Evaluation
B2   Therapeutic Exercise
B3   Transfer Training
B4   Home Program
B5   Gait Training
B6   Pulmonary Physical Therapy
B7   UltraSound
B8   Electrotherapy
B9   Prosthetic Training
B10   Fabrication of Temporary Gait Training Devices
B11   Muscle Re-education
B12   Management and Evaluation of a Patient Care Plan
B13–14 Reserved
B15* Other (Specify under orders)

Speech Therapy

C1   Evaluation
C2   Voice Disorders Treatments
C3   Speech Articulation Disorders Treatments
C4   Dysphagia Treatments
C5   Language Disorders Treatments

*Code that requires a more extensive descriptive narrative for physician's orders.

C6   Aural Rehabilitation
C7   Reserved
C8   Nonoral Communication
C9*   Other (Specify under orders)

Occupational Therapy

D1   Evaluation
D2   Independent Living/Daily Living Skills (ADL Training)
D3   Muscle Re-education
D4   Reserved
D5   Perceptual Motor Training
D6   Fine Motor Coordination
D7   Neuro-developmental Treatment
D8   Sensory Treatment
D9   Orthotics/Splinting
D10   Adaptive Equipment (fabrication and training)
D11* Other (Specify under orders)

Medical Social Services

E1   Assessment of Social and Emotional Factors
E2   Counseling for Long-Range Planning and Decision Making
E3   Community Resource Planning
E4*   Short-Term Therapy
E5   Reserved
E6*   Other (Specify under orders)

Home Health Aide

F1   Tub/Shower Bath
F2   Partial/Complete Bed Bath
F3   Reserved
F4   Personal Care
F5   Reserved
F6   Catheter Care
F7   Reserved
F8   Assist with Ambulation
F9   Reserved

*Code that requires a more extensive descriptive narrative for physician's orders.

F10   Exercises
F11   Prepare Meal
F12   Grocery Shop
F13   Wash Clothes
F14   Housekeeping
F15*   Other (Specify under orders)

- *C3. Speech Articulation Disorders Treatments*—Procedures and treatment for patients with impaired intelligibility (clarity) of speech—usually referred to as anarthria or dysarthria, and/or impaired ability to initiate, inhibit, and/or sequence speech sound muscle movements—usually referred to as apraxia/dyspraxia.
- *C4. Dysphagia Treatments*—Includes procedures designed to facilitate and restore a functional swallow.
- *C5. Language Disorders Treatments*—Includes procedures and treatment for patients with receptive and/or expressive aphasia/dysphasia, impaired reading comprehension, written language expression, and/or arithmetical processes.
- *C6. Aural Rehabilitation*—Procedures and treatments designed for patients with communication problems related to impaired hearing acuity.
- *C7. Reserved*
- *C8. Nonoral Communications*—Includes any procedures designed to establish a nonoral or augmentive communication system.
- *C9. Other (Specify under orders)*—Speech therapy services not included above. Specify service to be rendered under physician's orders (HCFA-485, Item 21).

*Code that requires a more extensive descriptive narrative for physician's orders.

Appendix D

Glossary

The following terms are related to medical conditions and management.

Acetylcholine. The neurotransmitter released at the synapses of parasympathetic nerves and at neuromuscular junctions. After relaying a nerve impulse, acetylcholine is rapidly broken down by the enzyme, cholinesterase.

Agranulocytosis. A disorder in which there is a severe acute deficiency of certain blood cells (neutrophils) as a result of damage to the bone marrow by toxic drugs or chemicals. It is characterized by fever, with ulceration of the mouth and throat, and may rapidly lead to prostration and death. Agranulocytosis can be a side effect of certain psychotropic drugs.

Akathisia. Restless overactivity, involuntary movements induced by antipsychotic drugs.

Akinesia. A loss of normal muscle tone or responsiveness.

Allergic reaction; Allergy. An undesirable response occurring in individuals producing antibodies that react with drugs. Allergic reactions may appear as skin rash, fever, painful joints, breathing difficulty, and collapse of circulation. Drug allergies can develop gradually or can appear suddenly. Some allergic reactions are life threatening.

Amenorrhea. Absence or stopping of the menstrual periods. Amenorrhea is a side effect of certain drugs and is a symptom of depression.

Amyotrophy. A progressive loss of muscle bulk associated with weakness of these muscles. It is a feature of chronic neuropathy. Amyotrophy combined with spasticity characterizes motor neuron disease.

Source: Adapted with permission by the Singular Publishing Group, Inc., D. Vogel and J. Carter, *The Effects of Drugs on Communication Disorders.*

Anaphylaxis. An abnormal reaction to a particular antigen in which histamine is released from the tissues and causes either local or widespread symptoms. An allergic attack is an example of localized anaphylaxis. Rarer, but much more serious, is anaphylactic shock in which widespread histamine release causes swelling, constrictions of the bronchioles, heart failure, circulatory collapse and, sometimes, death.

Aneurysm. A balloon-like swelling in the wall of an artery. Aneurysms within the brain can be congenital, and if they burst, they may cause a subarachnoid hemorrhage.

Antibodies. Blood proteins that combine with substances that are foreign to the body. Antibodies either can be protective or injurious. Protective antibodies destroy bacteria and neutralize toxins, while injurious antibodies, combined with foreign substances, cause allergic reactions.

Anticholinergics, anticholinergic drugs. Drugs that inhibit the action of acetylcholine. Side effects of anticholinergics include dry mouth, blurred vision, and dizziness. More serious side effects are impaired cognition, constipation, urinary retention, and precipitation of untreated glaucoma.

Anticholinesterase. A substance that inhibits the action of cholinesterase, the enzyme responsible for the breakdown of the neurotransmitter, acetylcholine. Anticholinesterase allows acetylcholine to continue transmitting nerve impulses.

Anticonvulsant. A drug that prevents or reduces the severity of seizures in various types of epilepsy. The choice of anticonvulsant is dictated by the type of seizure and the response to the drug. Some anticonvulsants are used for all types of seizures, others are type specific.

Antidepressant. A drug that alleviates the symptoms of depression. The most widely prescribed are the tricyclic antidepressants. Another main group of antidepressants are the MAO inhibitors; these have more severe side effects than the tricyclics.

Aplastic anemia. A disorder of white blood cell production.

Arrhythmia. A deviation from the normal rhythm (sinus rhythm) of the heart. Arrhythmias may be intermittent or continuous and may arise from various causes including the adverse effect of certain drugs.

Arthralgia. Pain in a joint without swelling or arthritis.

Asthenia. Weakness or loss of strength.

Astrocytoma. A brain tumor in which all grades of malignancy occur—from slow growing, with nearly normal cells, to rapidly growing, highly invasive tumors.

Ataxia. Unsteady gait with incoordination of movement. Ataxic (cerebellar) dysarthria may coexist with the unsteady gait.

Atrophy. The wasting away of a normally developed organ or tissue due to degeneration of cells.

Autism. A severe psychiatric disorder of childhood manifested by severe difficulties in communicating, forming relationships, developing language, and using abstract concepts.

Autoimmune disease. A disease thought to be caused by inflammation and destruction of tissues by the body's own antibodies.

Barbiturate. Drugs derived from barbituric acid that depress the activity of the central nervous system. Slow-acting barbiturates may be used to control seizures.

Benign. Description of a tumor that does not invade or destroy the tissue in which it originates. Benign tumors do not metastasize. Often the term "benign" is used to describe a tumor that is not cancerous.

Beta blocker. A drug that prevents stimulation of receptors of the nerves of the sympathetic nervous system and therefore decreases the activity of the heart. Beta blockers may be used to control abnormal heart rhythms, to treat angina, and to reduce high blood pressure.

Blood-brain barrier. The mechanism whereby the circulating blood is kept separate from the tissue fluids surrounding the brain cells.

Blood dyscrasia. An abnormal state of the blood, usually due to abnormal development or metabolism.

Bone marrow depression. Bone marrow is the tissue contained within the internal cavities of the bones. At birth, these cavities are filled with blood-forming tissue, but in later life the marrow in the limb bones is replaced by fat. Depression of bone marrow is a side effect of certain drugs.

Bradykinesia. A symptom of Parkinson's disease manifested by difficulty in initiating movements, slowness in executing movements, and an inability to make adjustments to posturing of the body.

Brand name. The registered trade name given to a drug by its manufacturer. The brand name designates that the drug is protected by a patent or copyright.

Bruise, contusion. An area of skin discoloration caused by the escape of blood from ruptured underlying vessels following injury. The drawing off of blood through a needle may be necessary to aid the healing of very severe bruises.

Bureau of Drugs. A division of the United Sates Food and Drug Administration responsible for the regulation of drugs available to patients. The efficacy of new drugs must be proven before the drugs can be prescribed by physicians.

Cause-effect relationship. A possible association between a drug and a side effect. Often it is not possible to establish that a drug is responsible for an effect. Cause-effect relationships are more likely to be established when the effect immediately follows the administration of the drug and when the adverse effect disappears after the drug is discontinued and reappears after subsequent use. In establishing cause-effect relationships, consideration must be given to progression of disease, the interval between the administration and a reaction to the drug, and the interaction between drugs if more than one is taken.

Chemotherapy. The prevention or treatment of a disease by the use of chemical substances. The term is restricted to drugs used to control cancer.

Clonic. Relating to or resembling clonus. The term is used to describe the rhythmic limb movements in epilepsy.

Compliance. The taking of medication as the prescriber intended. Conversely, noncompliance is not taking the medication as intended by the prescriber, whether consciously or through error or misunderstanding.

Contraindication. Any factor that makes it unwise to pursue a particular treatment. For example, a specific condition may be a contraindication against the use of a certain drug.

Craniotomy. Surgical removal of a portion of the skull to expose the cortex and meninges for inspection or biopsy. Craniotomy is performed to relieve excessive intracranial pressure, as in subdural hematoma.

Cushing's syndrome. A condition resulting from excess amounts of corticosteroid hormones in the body. Symptoms include weight gain, reddening of the face and neck, excess growth of body and facial hair, raised blood pressure, loss of mineral from bone (osteoporosis), raised blood glucose levels, and, sometimes, cognitive disturbances.

Demyelination. A process that selectively damages the myelin sheath in the nervous system. Affecting the nerve fibers supported by the myelin, demyelination may be the primary disorder, as in multiple sclerosis, or may occur secondary to brain injury or stroke.

Diaphoresis. The process of sweating, especially excessive sweating.

Diplopia. Double vision. The simultaneous awareness of two images of one object. Usually diplopia is due to a disturbance in the coordination of muscles that move the eye. Covering one eye will stop the diplopia.

Disease. A disorder with a specific cause and recognizable signs and symptoms. A bodily abnormality or failure to function normally, except when resulting directly from physical injury.

Disorientation. A state produced by loss of awareness of space, time, or person. Disorientation can be a consequence of drugs, anxiety, or organic disease.

Dispensary. A place where medicines are made up by a pharmacist and dispensed to patients.

Drug. A medicine used in medical practice. A chemical entity that provokes a specific response when it is placed in a biological system.

Drug class. A group of drugs similar in chemistry, method of action, and use. Drugs within the same class can produce similar beneficial effects and side effects. Significant variations may occur that allow the physician to choose a particular drug if certain beneficial actions are desired or certain side effects are to be minimized or avoided.

Gait. The manner in which a person walks. In neurological disease, the gait is often unsteady or uncoordinated. A staggering gait indicates alcohol or barbiturate intoxication or can be an indication of cerebellar disease.

Gamma-aminobutyric acid (GABA). An amino acid in the brain, where it acts as an inhibitory neurotransmitter.

Generic name. The official, common, or public name used to designate a specific drug by its principal active ingredients. Many drugs have no brand name. Generics, as a rule, are less expensive than brand name drugs and may be, but are not always, identical to a prescribed brand name drug.

Glioblastoma multiforme. An aggressive type of brain tumor. Its rapid enlargement destroys normal brain cells, with a progressive loss of function. The resultant raised intracranial pressure causes headache, vomiting, and drowsiness.

Glioma. A term frequently used for all tumors that arise in the central nervous system, including astrocytomas, oligodendrogliomas, and medulloblastomas. Tumors of low-grade malignancy produce symptoms by their pressure on surrounding structures. Those of high-grade malignancy may be invasive.

Granulocytopenia. A reduction of the number of granulocytes (a type of white cell) in the blood.

Hallucination. A false perception of something that is not really there. Hallucinations may be visual, auditory, tactile, or of taste or smell. They may be provoked by psychological illness, for example, schizophrenia, or by physical disorders involving the brain, for example, temporal lobe epilepsy or stroke; or they may be caused by drugs or sensory deprivation.

Hemorrhagic pancreatitis. Pancreatitis is an inflammation of the pancreas, a compound gland that lies beneath the stomach. In hemorrhagic pancreatitis, there is bleeding into the pancreas. Possible causes are gall stones or alcoholism.

Hepatitis. An inflammation of the liver caused by viruses, toxic substances, or immunological abnormalities.

Hepatotoxicity, hepatotoxic reaction. Damage or destruction to liver cells. Certain drugs can cause hepatotoxicity.

Hirsutism. The presence of coarse hair on the face, chest, upper back, or abdomen as a side effect of certain drugs.

Hypersensitivity. Overresponsiveness to drug action. Intolerance to even small doses. Some individuals who are allergic to a particular drug will be allergic to other drugs that are closely related in chemical composition (*see* **Drug Class**).

Hypnotic. A drug used primarily to induce sleep. Antihistamines, barbiturates, and benzodiazepines are classes of drugs that produce hypnotic effects.

Hypothermia. Accidental reduction of body temperature below the normal range in the absence of reflex actions, for example, shivering. Hypothermia occurs most often in infants and older persons. It can be a side effect of certain drugs.

Hypoxic-ischemic insult. A deficiency of oxygen in the tissues, leading to ischemic insult.

Iatrogenic. Description of a condition resulting from treatment, as either an unforeseen or inevitable side effect.

Idiopathic. A disease or condition the cause of which is unknown. Idiopathic diseases or conditions may arise spontaneously.

Immunosuppressant drug. A drug that reduces the body's resistance to infection and other foreign bodies by suppressing the immune system. Because immunity is lowered during treatment with immunosuppressants there is an increased risk of infection. Immunosuppressant drugs are used for treating chronic autoimmune diseases.

Injection. Introduction into the body of drugs or other fluids by means of a syringe. Usually these drugs, if taken orally, would be destroyed by the digestive process. Common routes for injection are intracutaneous (into the skin), subcutaneous (below the skin), intramuscular (into a muscle for slow absorption), and intravenous (into a vein for rapid absorption).

Insomnia. Inability to fall asleep or to remain asleep for an adequate length of time to eliminate tiredness. Insomnia may be associated with disease or may occur as a side effect of certain drugs.

Interaction. An unwanted change in the response to a drug that results when another drug is administered at the same time. Drug interactions can enhance the effect of either drug, reduce drug effectiveness, or produce a toxic response (*see* **Toxicity**).

Intervention study. A comparison of the outcome between two or more groups of patients that are deliberately subjected to different drug regimens. Patients in the control group have no active treatment. Patients in the experimental groups are subjected to active drug treatment. In a randomized controlled trial, all subjects are assigned randomly to control or experimental groups. Ideally, the study should be a double blind cross-over design in which neither the patient nor the experimenter assessing the outcome is aware of the group to which the patient has been assigned. In these studies in which two drugs or a drug and a placebo are administered, study patients exchange treatments after a prearranged period.

Jaundice. A yellow coloration of the skin and the white of the eyes that occurs when excessive bile pigments accumulate in the blood as a result of impaired liver function. Jaundice may be a sign of disease or a reaction to a particular drug.

Kayser-Fleischer ring. A brownish-yellow ring in the outer rim of the cornea of the eye caused by a deposit of copper granules. This sign is diagnostic of Wilson's disease. When well developed these rings may be seen by the naked eye, but if faint, they may be detected only by specialized ophthalmological examination.

Leukopenia. A reduction of the number of white blood cells (leukocytes) in the blood.

MAO Inhibitor. A drug that prevents the activity of the enzyme monoamine oxidase (MAO) in brain tissue and therefore affects mood. Their use may be restricted because of the severity of their side effects.

Medication. A substance administered by mouth, applied to the skin, or introduced into the body for the purpose of treatment.

Meningioma. A tumor arising from the meninges, the fibrous coverings of the brain and spinal cord.

Mitral valve prolapse. The mitral valve is located in the heart and consists of two flaps attached to the walls at the opening between the left atrium and the left ventricle. It allows the blood to pass through the atrium to the ventricle but prevents backward flow. Mitral valve prolapse refers to a downward displacement of the valve from its normal position and usually is the result of weakening of its supporting tissues.

Mydriasis. A widening of the pupil that occurs normally in dim light. The most common causes of prolonged mydriasis are drug therapy or injuries to the eye.

Neoplasm (of the brain). An abnormal multiplication of brain cells. This forms edema that compresses or destroys healthy brain cells and, because the skull is rigid, increases pressure on the brain.

Nephritis. Inflammation of the kidney. Also referred to as Bright's disease.

Nephrotic syndrome. A condition in which, due to edema, there is great loss of protein in the urine, reduced levels of albumin in the blood, and generalized swelling of the tissues.

Neuroblastoma. A malignant tumor composed of embryonic nerve cells.

Neurofibromatosis. A congenital disease typified by numerous benign tumors growing from the fibrous coverings of nerves. Tumors may occur in the spinal canal, where they may press on the spinal cord. Pigmented patches on the skin are found in a large number of cases. This condition is also known as von Recklinghausen's disease.

Neuroleptic malignant syndrome. A rare, serious, potentially fatal reaction to antipsychotic drugs.

Neurotransmitter. A chemical substance released from nerve endings to transmit impulses across synapses to other muscles, nerves, or glands.

Optic neuropathy. Neuropathy is any disease of the peripheral nerves, usually causing weakness and numbness. Optic neuropathy refers to disease of the optic nerve and, often, is diagnostic of multiple sclerosis.

Orphan drug. A drug used for treating relatively rare conditions and that thus has no potential for making a profit for the drug manufacturer. Many requirements of the Food and Drug Administration are omitted. There are more than 100 orphan drugs.

318 THE SPEECH-LANGUAGE PATHOLOGIST IN HOME HEALTH CARE

318 THE SPEECH-LANGUAGE PATHOLOGIST IN HOME HEALTH CARE

Orthostatic hypotension (Postural hypotension). Low blood pressure related to body position or posture. The blood pressure may be normal when lying down, but upon sitting or standing sudden sensations of dizziness, lightheadedness, and feeling faint are experienced, resulting in the quick return to the lying down position. The condition is due to inadequate oxygen supply and, therefore, inadequate blood flow to the brain. This results in an abnormal delay in the rise of blood pressure that occurs as the body adjusts the circulation to the upright position.

Over-the-counter (OTC) drugs (Nonprescription drugs). Drugs that may be purchased without prescription. These products should be regarded as medicines that can interact with prescription or other OTC drugs.

Overdose. More than the optimal dosage resulting from a variety of sources. Overdose can result from the accumulation of prescribed daily doses of a drug or can occur with accidental ingestion of drugs, for example, by children or by adults with suicidal intention.

Palilalia. A disorder in which a word is rapidly and involuntarily repeated. It occurs in Gilles de la Tourette syndrome and other disorders of the extrapyramidal system.

Palliative. A medicine or procedure that gives temporary relief from symptoms but does not cure the underlying disease.

Pallidectomy. A neurosurgical procedure designed to destroy or modify the effects of the globus pallidus. This procedure is used for relief of Parkinson's disease and other conditions in which involuntary movements are prominent.

Paradoxical reaction. An unexpected drug response that is inconsistent with known pharmacology. These reactions may be due to individual sensitivity and appear to be more common in children and older persons.

Paraparesis. Weakness of both legs, resulting from disease of the nervous system.

Parenteral. Administration of a drug through other than oral administration; for example, by injection.

Pedal edema. Swelling of the foot.

Pharmacodynamics. The interaction of drugs with cells.

Pharmacokinetics. The process of absorption, distribution, metabolism, and excretion of a drug.

Pharmacology. The science of development and use of medicines, including the composition of medicines and their actions in animals and humans.

Pharmacy. The preparation and dispensing of drugs. A place registered to dispense medicines.

Phenylketonuria. A congenital defect of protein metabolism that causes excessive amounts of the amino acid phenylalanine in the blood. The condition causes damage to the nervous system and leads to severe mental retardation.

The responsible gene is recessive, so a child is affected only if both parents are carriers of the defective gene.

Photophobia. An abnormal intolerance of light, in which exposure to light causes intense discomfort to the eyes. Tight contraction of the eyelids and other reactions may be used to avoid the light. Photophobia may be associated with dilation of the pupils as a reaction to certain drugs.

Placebo. A drug that is ineffective but may relieve symptoms because the patient believes it will. New drugs are tested against placebos in clinical trials. The placebo response is one that occurs even in the absence of any pharmacologically active substance.

Plasmapheresis. The method of removing a quantity of plasma from a patient's blood. After the plasma is removed, the blood cells are transfused back into the patient.

Polypharmacy. Treatment with more than one type of medicine.

Prescription. A written direction from a medical practitioner to a pharmacist for preparing and dispensing a drug.

Prognosis. Assessment of the future course and outcome of a patient's condition, based on knowledge of the outcome of the condition in other patients. The patient's general health, age, and sex are considered in the prognosis.

Psychosis. A severe psychiatric illness in which the patient loses contact with reality.

Ptosis. The drooping of the upper eyelid, for which there are several causes, including a disorder of the oculomotor nerve or a widespread fatigable weakness.

Radiotherapy. The treatment of a disease with penetrating radiation, which may be produced by machines or radioactive isotopes. Beams of radiation may be directed at a diseased organ from a distance, or radioactive material in the form of needles, wires, or pellets may be implanted in the body. Many forms of cancer are destroyed by radiation; however, radiation can damage normal tissues.

Resting tremor. A rhythmic to and fro movement of the extremity.

Rigidity. Increased resistance to passive movements of a limb that is present throughout the range of movement.

Sepsis. Destruction of tissues by disease-causing bacteria or their toxins.

Side effect. An undesirable response to a drug. The majority of side effects are minor annoyances and inconveniences; but some are counterproductive in disease management, and some are potentially dangerous.

Sign. An indication of a disease or a disorder noticed by someone other than the patient, often by the physician.

Spasm. A sustained muscle contraction.

Spasticity. Resistance to the passive movement of a limb that is maximal at the beginning of the movement, giving way as more pressure is applied. Spasticity is a symptom of damage to the corticospinal tracts in the brain or spinal cord, and usually is accompanied by weakness in the affected limb.

Stereotaxic technique. A surgical procedure in which a deep-seated area in the brain is operated on after its position has been established accurately by three-dimensional measurements. The operation may be performed using an electrical current or by heat, cold, or mechanical techniques.

Stupor. A condition of near unconsciousness with no apparent mental activity and reduced ability to respond to stimulation.

Subarachnoid hemorrhage. Bleeding into the subarachnoid space surrounding the brain that causes severe headache with stiffness of the neck. The usual source is a cerebral aneurysm.

Symptom. An indication of a disease or disorder noticed by the patient, him- or herself.

Symptomatology. Collectively, the symptoms of a disease.

Syncope. Fainting, that is, loss of consciousness induced by a temporarily insufficient flow of blood to the brain. Syncope may be caused by an emotional shock, by standing for prolonged periods, by injury with profuse bleeding, or it may be a side effect of a drug. An attack comes on gradually with lightheadedness, sweating, and blurred vision. Typically, recovery is prompt, without any persisting ill effects from the syncope itself.

Tablet. A small disk containing one or more drugs. Tablets are made by compressing a powdered form of the drugs and are taken orally.

Tachycardia. An increase in heart rate to above normal. Tachycardia may be produced by arrhythmias.

Tardive dyskinesia. A drug-induced disorder of the nervous system occurring after long-term treatment with psychotropic drugs.

Thalamotomy. Surgery in which a lesion is made in a precise area of the thalamus. Thalamotomy has been used to control psychiatric symptoms of severe anxiety (psychosurgery), in which case, the lesion is made in the dorsomedial nucleus of the thalamus that connects with the frontal lobe. Thalamotomy has been used to control symptoms of Parkinson's disease.

Thrombocytopenia. A reduction in the number of platelets in the blood that may result from failure of platelet production or excessive destruction of platelets. Thrombocytopenia may result in bleeding into the skin, spontaneous bruising, and prolonged bleeding after injury.

Thrombophlebitis. Inflammation of the wall of a vein that may lead to secondary thrombosis occurring within the affected segment of the vein.

Thymoma. A benign or malignant tumor of the thymus gland.

Thyrotropin-releasing hormone (TRH). A hormone-like substance from the hypothalamus that acts on the anterior pituitary gland to stimulate the release of thyroid-stimulating hormone.

Tic. A repeated involuntary movement.

Tolerance. Reduced responsiveness to a drug. Certain medicines or dosages are not effective. A change in the drug or dosage becomes necessary. Side effects may occur, then disappear, during continuous use of a drug.

Toxicity. Having a poisonous effect; potentially lethal. A toxic drug has the potential for dangerously impairing body functions or damaging body tissues. Usually, the larger the dose, the greater the toxicity; however, some drugs can produce toxic reactions even when used in small doses.

Transient ischemic attack (TIA). A sudden, rapid onset of a focal neurologic deficit caused by a cerebrovascular disease. The deficit lasts less than 24 hours, reverting completely to normal.

Tremor. A rhythmic alternating movement.

SUGGESTED READING

Editors of Market House Books, Ltd. (1990). *The Bantam medical dictionary*. New York: Bantam Books.

Long, J.W. (1993). *The essential guide to prescription drugs*. New York: Harper Collins.

Meyer, M.E. (1993). *Coping with medications*. San Diego, CA: Singular Publishing Group.

APPENDIX E

General Abbreviations

po	per os (by mouth)
rect.	rectal
supp	suppository
qd	every day
qod	every other day
q	every
X	times
bid	two times per day
tid	three times per day
qid	four times per day
q mo	every month
q wk	every week
H.S.	hour of sleep
noc	night
pc	post cibum (after meals)
ac	ante cibum (before meals)
q a.m.	every morning
q p.m.	every night
I & O	intake and output
I & D	incision and drainage
amb	ambulatory
BP	blood pressure
B.R.	bedrest
B.R.P.	bathroom privileges

Courtesy of National Home Caring Council Foundation for Hospice and Homecare, Washington, DC.

w/c	wheelchair
SOB	shortness of breath
T.C.	telephone call
c̄	with
s̄	without
i.e.	that is
e.g.	for example
VS	vital signs: BP, blood pressure
ROM	range of motion
Tx	treatment
DX	diagnosis
Rehab Pot	rehabilitation potential
UA	urinalysis
K	potassium
Na	sodium
DC	discontinue
Fx	fracture
ADL	activities of daily living
TPR	temperature, pulse and respirations
ā	before
p̄	after
DSD	dry sterile dressing

Diagnostic Categories

ASHD	Arteriosclerotic heart disease
CHF	Congestive heart failure
CRF	Chronic renal failure
CVA	Cerebro vascular accident
CA	Cancer
COPD	Chronic obstructive pulmonary disease
CP	Cerebral palsy
ALS	Amyotrophic lateral sclerosis
MD	Muscular dystrophy
MS	Multiple sclerosis
MI	Myocardial infarction
TIA	Transient ischemic attack
Quad	Quadriplegic
Para	Paraplegic
Hemi	Hemiplegic

CNS   Central nervous system
Mets   Metastatic

Professional Personnel

VN   Visiting nurse
RPT   Registered physical therapist
OTR   Registered occupational therapist
S.T.   Speech therapist
R.D.   Registered dietitian
MSW   Medical social worker
HCA   Home care aide
Sup   Supervisor
Nsg   Nursing

Index

denial of payment, 146–147
guidelines, 144–148
methods, 143–144
review of service, 146–147
speech-language pathology
coverage, 145–146
speech-language pathology
services, 196–199
Medication
defined, 317
older patient, 67–69
adverse drug reaction, 67–68
compliance, 67
drug interaction, 68
Meningioma, defined, 317
Mitral valve prolapse, defined, 317
Mobility, 93
Money management, 92
Mydriasis, defined, 317

N

National Association of Home Health
Agencies, 9
National Homecaring Council, 9
National League for Nursing, 9
Needle, 88–89
Nephritis, defined, 317
Nephrotic syndrome, defined, 317
Networking, 154
Neuroblastoma, defined, 317
Neurofibromatosis, defined, 317
Neuroleptic malignant syndrome,
defined, 317
Neurological integrity, assessment,
62–63
Neurologist, referral, 30
Neurotransmitter, defined, 317
Nonhemispheric disorder, Medicare,
141–142
Nonprescription drug, defined, 318

Not-for-profit organization, 4–5
Nutritional health, 91
assessment, 60–62

O

Occupational exposure, defined, 87
Occupational Safety and Health
Administration, bloodborne
pathogen standard, 85–90
Occupational therapist, dysphagia, 37
Older Americans Act, 137
Older patient
assessment, methodological
concerns, 65–67
competency assessment, 252–253
medication, 66–69
adverse drug reaction, 67–68
compliance, 67
drug interaction, 68
Operation Restore Trust, 287–288
Optic neuropathy, defined, 317
Oral-facial muscle, manual muscle
testing, 69–71, 248–249
Orphan drug, defined, 317
Orthostatic hypotension, defined,
318
Outcome goal, plan of care,
102–103
Outcome measure, 233
Outcome-based quality improvement,
217, 231–234
end-result outcome, 232–233
focus, 232
outcome measure, 233
Outcome and Assessment
Information Set (OASIS),
233–234
Outcome and Assessment
Information Set (OASIS),
217, 233–234